Language Strategies for Bilingual Families

PARENTS' AND TEACHERS' GUIDES

Series Editor: Colin Baker, *Bangor University, UK*

This series provides immediate advice and practical help on topics where parents and teachers frequently seek answers. Each book is written by one or more experts in a style that is highly readable, non-technical and comprehensive. No prior knowledge is assumed: a thorough understanding of a topic is promised after reading the appropriate book.

Full details of all the books in this series and of all our other publications can be found on http://www.multilingual-matters.com, or by writing to Multilingual Matters, St Nicholas House, 31–34 High Street, Bristol BS1 2AW, UK.

Language Strategies for Trilingual Families

Parents' Perspectives

Andreas Braun and Tony Cline

MULTILINGUAL MATTERS
Bristol • Buffalo • Toronto

Library of Congress Cataloging in Publication Data
A catalog record for this book is available from the Library of Congress.
Braun, Andreas, (Linguist)
Language Strategies for Trilingual Families: Parents' Perspectives/Andreas Braun and Tony Cline.
Parents' and Teachers' Guides: 17
Includes bibliographical references and index.
1. Multilingualism in children. 2. Multicultural education. 3. Education, Bilingual.
4. Multilingualism. I. Cline, Tony, author. II. Title.
P115.2.B73 2014
404'.2085–dc23 2013036370

British Library Cataloguing in Publication Data
A catalogue entry for this book is available from the British Library.

ISBN-13: 978-1-78309-115-7 (hbk)
ISBN-13: 978-1-78309-114-0 (pbk)

Multilingual Matters
UK: St Nicholas House, 31-34 High Street, Bristol BS1 2AW, UK.
USA: UTP, 2250 Military Road, Tonawanda, NY 14150, USA.
Canada: UTP, 5201 Dufferin Street, North York, Ontario M3H 5T8, Canada.

The policy of Multilingual Matters/Channel View Publications is to use papers that are natural, renewable and recyclable products, made from wood grown in sustainable forests. In the manufacturing process of our books, and to further support our policy, preference is given to printers that have FSC and PEFC Chain of Custody certification. The FSC and/or PEFC logos will appear on those books where full certification has been granted to the printer concerned.

Typeset by R. J. Footring Ltd, Derby
Printed and bound in Great Britain by CPI Antony Rowe

Contents

Figures and Tables

Figures

Tables

Acknowledgements

We would like to thank all the trilingual families who gave their precious time in research interviews, emails and web forums to provide us with a snapshot of their trilingual experience. Without their help this book would not have been possible.

1 Trilingualism and Multilingualism: An Overview

Introduction

In the world today, with increasing globalisation, many more people move, work, live and marry across borders. More children are born to parents who, between them, speak two or three languages or even more. The European Union alone has 24 official languages, and in fact the number of official languages is growing not just in Europe but also in Asia, Africa, North and South America and Australia. This has created new forms of trilingualism and, with them, new linguistic and cultural challenges for parents who have different nationalities and native languages. When children grow up in circumstances where the people around them can speak three or more languages, their parents face a question that they may not be prepared for: how can the children be helped to make the most of the complex heritage of languages and cultures that are available to them? Most of us learn our strategies for parenting from our own parents. But parents who have themselves grown up in monolingual or even bilingual settings will have no ready models for trilingual parenting.

This book aims to help parents and professionals to tackle the specific challenges faced by trilingual families with children. Books on trilingualism and multilingualism tend to focus on young children. They address questions such as when and how children acquire three languages and in what circumstances they use them. Here, in addition, we will consider the position of the parents in trilingual families. They have received less attention, but their role is crucial. Their practices and decisions will determine how far the children benefit from the opportunities they have for becoming trilingual. We will report how some parents have responded to the challenge, and hope that this will provide a stimulus for readers to reflect on the situations they face.

Much of what has been written about trilingualism has drawn on concepts that were developed in the study of bilingualism. But, while there are some overlaps, the ways in which languages and cultural traditions interact in trilingual families are more complex. Because there are more languages involved, language maintenance is more difficult, and the situation as a whole is more challenging. So there is a growing demand for information and advice on trilingualism (and multilingualism more generally) from parents who feel that what they read and are told about bilingualism does not fully answer the questions they have about the development of their own children. This led many volunteers to take part in the research study on which this book is mainly based, a project carried out by Andreas, who interviewed parents and some teenagers in 35 trilingual families in England and 35 families in Germany (see the next section for more information). Our ultimate goal is to provide an account that will help other parents in trilingual families to review their options and make informed choices. Many parents will want to pass on all the languages in their repertoire to their children, but some will not. We will discuss the reasons that are given for different choices and enable readers to evaluate the options for themselves. Thus the book addresses four broad questions:

- How will parents' competence in their home languages and the community language influence their decision to use those languages with their children?
- What strategies do parents employ at home and outside in order to foster particular languages with their children?
- How are parents' choices influenced by their linguistic and cultural backgrounds?
- What impact do the beliefs and attitudes of members of the extended family and other people have on trilingual families' language practices?

Other issues that were frequently mentioned by parents and that we cover in the book include:

- uncertainty about when to introduce a third language to a child;
- being consistent about using particular languages at home and outside;
- mixing languages;
- developing a minority language;
- difficulties at school;
- children's sense of identity.

Our Sources

The main source for the book was Andreas's interviews conducted with parents in trilingual families living in England and Germany. Most participants could speak English, except some families in Germany where the interviews were conducted in German, which were translated by Andreas. The majority of these parents were in their 30s; their average age was about 38 years, although the youngest parent was 18 and the oldest 56. The parents had a total of 46 nationalities and spoke over 40 different native languages between them. The largest number had British or German nationality, but there were also significant numbers with Finnish, Russian, Italian, US-American and French nationality. While most came from a white European ethnic background, there was also a representation of a range of other ethnic minorities.

Questions were addressed to the parents together where both were available for the interview. Occasionally teenage children joined in the meeting and were asked some questions too. The children had an average age of around seven years, slightly older in England on average and slightly younger in Germany. Because the research concerned parents in trilingual families and the social and linguistic effects of their language use with their children when they are still living at home, young people in the families over the age of 15 years were not included in our discussions. All trilingual families had the potential of using at least three languages between the community and their home. The interviews with the parents established their general background and explored their language background and their use of languages in the home in detail. They also covered issues relating to cultural practices and cultural identity. These themes will be discussed in later chapters.

In addition to the interview study, we have also drawn on approximately 150 contributions to an internet forum about trilingualism that has been online for some years (www.trilingualism.org) and on more than 250 anonymous emails. (The names of all participants in this book have been changed, in order to protect their anonymity.) For example, Abelena, a Mexican mother living in England, said: 'I would love to participate in your survey, and in turn learn more about how to facilitate my son's acquisition of these languages'. Oliva, a US-American mother living in Germany, said: 'Please also keep me informed on the results of your study. I think that there is a big need for the study on trilingualism.' Thus the content of the book has been informed by an analysis of what parents had to say in research interviews, anonymous emails and contributions to the web forum in the light of the current literature. That analysis focused on how adults and children communicate in trilingual families, on the factors that influence parents' choices around the use of the languages available to them and on how three or more possible languages are used in different settings.

Terminology

This is a field where different writers often use the same term in quite different ways. This short paragraph lists some of the terms that appear frequently in this book. We are concerned with *trilingual families*, that is, families in which the parents are in a position to provide their children with two native home languages in addition to the community languag; thus, between community and home, three languages are available. In this book we employ the term *community language* to refer to the language that is spoken in the wider community and neighbourhood in which a trilingual family lives. The terms *native language*, *heritage language* and *minority language* are used interchangeably to refer to one, two or three of the parents' languages which they acquired as native languages in the society in which they were living when they were young (i.e. in their formative years). The term *home languages* refers to the parents' native languages as a unit. It can also include the community language if one or both parents speak it as a native language. The terms *monolingual* and *bilingual* are used to describe individuals who have one or two native languages. *Multilingual* and *multilingualism* are used as general terms for a situation in which speakers are not just bilingual but show a mastery of three or more languages.

Pinpointing Family Language Background

The first step for any parent reading this book is to identify the family's language background. This is because the language strategies that we employ and the ways in which we use our languages change depending on who speaks which languages in the family and how many languages they speak individually and collectively. For example, a parent who speaks only one native language has different concerns from a parent who speaks two or three native languages. In order clarify family background, we have developed a framework for categorising multilingual families into three groups. All of the parents who fit in this framework have the potential to bring up their children to speak three or more native languages, but how they might do it and what factors may influence them will vary according to their language backgrounds. Figure 1.1 presents a series of questions that helps to determine the 'type' of multilingual family.

Families in the first trilingual group comprise monolingual parents who live in a country where their native languages are not the community language. They speak different native languages, and neither of them learned as a child the community language of the country where they now live. This group is the subject of Chapter 3. Examples include:

- Gerd speaks German as his native language and Säde, his wife, speaks Finnish. Both moved to England as adults for educational purposes before they met. They married in England and are bringing up their children there. This has created the opportunity for their children to learn three languages.
- Pietro, who is in his 40s, grew up in Italy. He and his Iranian wife, Afareen, had been living together for 10 years when they moved to England because of their work situation. Pietro spoke Italian as his native language, while Afareen spoke Persian-Farsi. They now both speak English fluently, as do their children.
- Adrijana is a native speaker of Serbo-Croatian and her husband, Anatoly, speaks Russian. They live in the USA, where they speak their respective native languages with their 14-month-old daughter. The parents communicate in English with each other and they plan to start introducing some English to their child a year before she starts going to a nursery.

Families in the second group (see Chapter 4) have at least one bilingual parent. A number of different language constellations are possible. They include families where one parent speaks one native language and the other parent two native languages, and also families where both parents speak two native languages. These may include the community language. Sometimes both parents are bilingual with the same linguistic background, but neither of them speaks the community language as a native language. The result is that their two shared languages plus the community language create a trilingual background for their children. Examples include:

- Adelina and Axel live in Germany. She speaks Italian and English as her native languages, while he speaks the community language, German, as a native language.

What is your background? A tool for diagnostic self-analysis

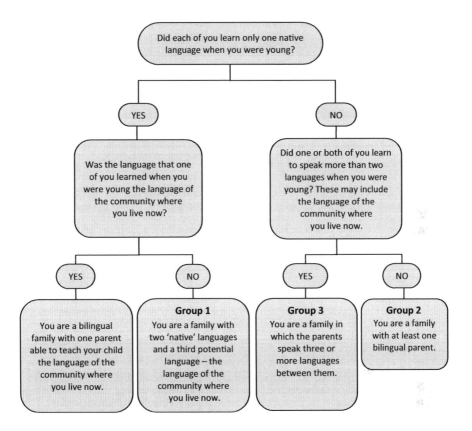

Figure 1.1 'Language background' tool

- Odval and Chuluun live in Germany. They both grew up with the same two native languages, Russian and Mongolian. Both parents were already adults when they moved to the host country to study at a university, where they learnt the community language as an additional language. Thus, in addition to their two native languages, German was available to the family when the children were born.
- Tereixa and Alfonso, who are both bilingual in Galician and Spanish, live in the French-speaking part of Switzerland. As parents they speak Galician with each other. They are expecting a child in a few weeks' time. Tereixa plans to speak only Galician to the child, whereas Alfonso intends to use Spanish. The social environment outside the home will be French-speaking.

Family members in the third group (see Chapter 5) speak three languages between them. Often, one or both parents are trilingual, although there are a number of other possible language constellations. Examples include:

- Anne and Michael live in England. She speaks Finnish, Swedish and English as native languages, while he speaks only English. To their child they speak only English, neglecting the mother's other two native languages.
- Irena left Lithuania for Germany 10 years ago with her parents. Gvidas came from Lithuania two years later to study and work in Germany with the intention of staying. Some years later they met and married in Germany. They both speak Russian and Lithuanian as native languages. In addition, Irena speaks German on a native level too, because she acquired it in Germany when she was still a girl. Gvidas speaks Lithuanian and Irena Russian with their young child, while German is the language of the community. However, Gvidas finds it increasingly hard to use Lithuanian because relatives around mainly speak Russian or German with the child.
- Sheker speaks Kazak and Russian as well as German and English and her husband, Adamo, speaks Italian, Spanish and French. The parents are very unsure about which and how many languages to use with their child. Adamo thinks he should refrain from using Spanish and French and use only Italian with his child.

An Outline of the Book

Each of the three main chapters focuses on one of these family groups. Some parents reading this book may wish to concentrate on the chapter that covers their specific language situation (as indicated from Figure 1.1). The chapters all cover four complementary themes:

- how parents decide to use languages with their children;
- languages at school;
- languages and the extended family;
- our languages and our cultures.

(a) How parents decide to use languages with their children

This is the fundamental issue that the book sets out to address. A key factor that influences language use is, of course, the language competence of the parents. That has been identified as the major reason for parents deciding whether or not to use a certain language with their children. There are exceptions. For example, some parents use a community language at home even though it is not their own preferred language, because they believe it will help their children to have a head start at school if they are exposed regularly to the language of the school in advance. With the same end in view, other parents employ a nanny who speaks the community language or enrol their children in nurseries at a very young age. Parents may alternatively adopt a deliberate strategy that is designed to enhance their children's command of their native languages rather than the community language. For example, they may each use one of their own native languages with the children in what is known as the OPOL method – One Parent One Language (also called One Person One Language). In the families briefly described in the previous section, Andrijana and Anatoly in Group 1, Tereixa and Alfonso in Group 2, and Irena and Gvidas in Group 3 were using the OPOL method when they were interviewed.

- In what ways may parents' language competence in the community language and in their native languages influence their family language practices?
- How useful is the OPOL method for different groups of trilingual families?

(b) Languages at school

This section of each chapter looks at the families' language practices in relation to their children's schooling. The settings that are examined include nurseries, preschools, primary schools, international schools and part-time supplementary schools. Parents are often very concerned about the effect that attendance at mainstream schools and nurseries may have on their children's use and maintenance of home languages. As soon as young children leave the 'safe' language environment of the home, they are liable to resort to the community language for vocabulary acquired at school which they would like to use at home. Some parents see this as an additional asset, while others emphasise the threat it poses to the children's use of their parents' native languages. Franciszek, a British/Polish father living in England, said:

> Sometimes if you wanted to speak the home language [Polish] with the child, the child would refuse because all their friends were using English. That started since they started going to school, age of four to five.

Some commentators have highlighted a lack of balance, as the home languages of multilingual families are overpowered by the influence of the community language in the school context. The aim of this section in each chapter is to investigate the influence of nurseries and schools on the maintenance of home languages in trilingual families from different language backgrounds. We show how some parents choose educational establishments that will support their children's acquisition of either the community language or selected home languages.

The global importance of the English language, in particular within education, and its effect on parents' use of their native languages is an additional focus of this section. Some parents perceive the high cultural status of English and its economic value in the workplace as worth seeking for their children, even at the expense of the maintenance of less widely used heritage languages from their own youth. But others see the dominant position of English as a threat to the balanced trilingualism that they would like their children to achieve. So we examine the high status of the English language in education in terms of its possible interference with the maintenance of home languages in multilingual families. Among the questions considered in this section of different chapters are:

- How does the linguistic milieu in nurseries, schools and other communal establishments (formal and informal) affect parents' decisions about the use of languages with their children?
- What educational strategies do parents employ in order to foster the community language and/or their home languages with their children?

(c) Languages and the extended family

In this section of each chapter we examine such issues as the influence of the extended family (e.g. grandparents, aunts, uncles, cousins) on trilingual families' language use with their children. What difference does it make when grandparents and other relatives live in the same country as the potentially trilingual family? What difference does it make when they live overseas and do not speak the community language with which their grandchildren are growing up? How is the outcome affected by parents' anxieties and their social ties and the attitudes of those close to them? It is necessary to distinguish between the three family language groups. For example, parents in Group 1 families have a monolingual language background and their parents are usually monolingual as well. This means that most of these grandparents would not be able to communicate with their grandchildren if the parents did not use their heritage languages with their children. The parents in a trilingual Group 1 family in Germany were asked to comment on their language choice. Patrick, who was 24 years old and originally from Ireland, worked as a businessman in Germany. His 31-year-old wife, Adriana, who was Portuguese, worked as a skilled professional. They had two boys, aged two years and one year, who were being brought up trilingually, with English and Portuguese at home and German elsewhere. When Adriana was asked why they used their respective native languages with their children, she answered:

> For both of us the same reason. None of our parents speak a foreign language and we want our children to be able to communicate with their grandparents. Furthermore we can't speak perfect German, which would not be nice if the children learnt broken German from us. I think they will learn it from friends, neighbours and in kindergarten.

Parents in Group 2 or Group 3 families, on the other hand, speak at least two native languages and so do most grandparents. Parents in these language groups are not as motivated as Group 1 parents to use all their native languages with their children. So in this section of each chapter we explore questions which we expect to be answered differently according to a family's language background:

- In what ways do grandparents and other relatives influence trilingual families' language practices?
- How can grandparents play a part in the maintenance of heritage languages?

(d) Our languages and our cultures

This section of Chapter 3–5 examines cultural issues and their effect on children's trilingual development. We consider the cultural factors that influence parents' use of languages with their children. That is affected by the way in which they identify themselves with the cultural traditions, customs and values that are attached to their native languages. Do cultural traditions always impact on parents' use of languages, or does language play a key role only when it is a core component of a culture? For parents from some types of language background, other markers, such as religion or ethnicity, may be the key factors, with language playing only a minor role in their sense of cultural identity. That is not true for Adela from Spain and Dirk from Germany, parents in a Group 1 family living in England, who each speak only one native language, which they associate strongly with their original cultural background:

Adela: Well, for me it's extremely important that [Mike, their son] understands and speaks Spanish because it's part of my identity and I want him to be part of that identity too.

Dirk: Exactly, yes. Yes, I think I don't have anything to add. It's part of my identity where I come from. In order to understand who I am, you need to understand the language as well.

We will also consider these issues in this section of the chapters on Group 2 and Group 3 families. Their different backgrounds and associated cultural traditions may create a totally different situation from the one described by Group 1 families. So in this section of each chapter we again explore questions which might be answered differently according to a family's language background:

- How do parents' perceptions of their cultural background affect their decisions on language use with their children in trilingual families?
- Are parents' different language backgrounds reflected in different cultural practices in their families?

Attitudes to Multilingualism in Society

It is often argued that children's development of bilingual or trilingual language proficiency is discouraged in some mainly monolingual societies because of the high social status of the principal language. In such countries politicians and even educationists often try to replace minority languages with the majority language. This leads to language uniformity taking precedence over language diversity. Monolingual people often think that language differences keep nations and people apart. Thus voters in many states of the USA have voted for English to be the sole official language, despite the existence of a sizeable minority of native speakers of Spanish and of Indian tribal languages. Proponents of English there argue that having only one official language for government, education and communication keeps the country together. There are also many countries which have a long history of official bilingualism, such as Finland, Kenya or the Republic of Ireland. But even in these countries one language is often dominant. It is also true that in countries such as Belgium, Spain, Ukraine, Lithuania and Latvia languages have become a symbolic and practical emblem of division. In such circumstances, the factors involved go beyond language and communication. Shifts in the use of languages express changes in the relative socioeconomic status of groups of speakers, and changes in cultural and religious beliefs and practices, as well as simple demographic change.

At the time when the families who are featured in this book were interviewed, there were more people speaking languages other than English at home in England and more people speaking languages other than German at home in Germany than there had ever been in the past. In Germany, according to the 2011 census, almost 10% of adult residents had a home language other than German. The largest linguistic minority spoke Turkish, followed by speakers of Italian, Polish, Greek and Russian (see Table 1.1). Between 2010 and 2012 the number of immigrants from Spain and Greece has more than doubled because of the economic crisis in those countries. The German census defines an immigrant as a person who possesses a non-German passport. Dual nationality or citizenship may be allowed only under special circumstances in Germany.

Table 1.1 Top eight minority nationalities in Germany (2011 census)

	Nationality	Number of people (% of total population)
1	Turkish	1,607,161 (1.96%)
2	Italian	520,159 (0.64%)
3	Polish	468,481 (0.57%)
4	Greek	283,684 (0.35%)
5	Croatian	223,014 (0.27%)
6	Serbian	197,984 (0.24%)
7	Russian	195,310 (0.24%)
8	Austrian	175,926 (0.21%)
	Total population of Germany	81,830,839

Source: Statistisches Bundesamt (www.destatis.de).

Table 1.2 Top eight countries for non-UK born residents in England and Wales (2011 census)

	Country of birth	Number of people (% of total population)
1	India	694,148 (1.24%)
2	Poland	579,121 (1.03%)
3	Pakistan	482,137 (0.86%)
4	Republic of Ireland	407,357 (0.73%)
5	Germany	273,564 (0.49%)
6	Bangladesh	211,500 (0.38%)
7	Nigeria	191,183 (0.34%)
8	South Africa	191,023 (0.34%)
	Total population of England and Wales	56,075,912

Source: Office for National Statistics (www.ons.gov.uk).

The UK census in 2011 showed similar figures (see Table 1.2): about 4 million people (8%) said that English was not their first language, while 13% (7.5 million) were born outside the UK; in 2001 the figures had been 9% (4.6 million). The number of people in the UK speaking Polish had shown a particularly dramatic increase following expansion of the European Union (EU) in 2004 to include Poland. According to the 2011 census, more than half a million people in England and Wales identified Polish as their main language, which was a nine-fold increase compared with 2001. The UK 2011 census defined an international migrant as a person born outside the UK.

Thus the language profiles of Germany and England have changed radically from the traditional image of two mainly monolingual societies. But the addition of many new communities of speakers has not had a substantial impact on general perceptions of language in either country. Leading politicians in both countries have spoken passionately in favour of new groups adopting the majority language. For example, in December 2012 the Labour Party leader in the UK, Ed Miliband, said:

> We can only converse if we can speak the same language. So if we are going to build one nation, we need to start with everyone in Britain knowing how to speak English. We should expect that of people that come here. We will work together as a nation far more effectively when we can always talk together. (*Guardian*, 2012)

To date, there has been no challenge to the dominance of English as the main language of the UK or to German as the main language of Germany.

It would be wrong, however, to suggest that the main challenges parents face in trilingual families arise from the ignorance and hostility of others. When parents from socially privileged backgrounds in England and Germany were interviewed, many of them were less concerned about hostility in the community and more worried about practical problems. Their children's trilingual development had often lost momentum, but not mainly because of negative social attitudes. For example, Ingrid, who is German, and her South African husband, Dakarai, reported on their experience in Germany:

Dakarai: A lot of people say: 'You are very lucky to have different languages'.
Ingrid: With immigrants it's different, like Armenians, Russians, Polish. With my husband it's different because he looks like a German and speaks very good German and some are surprised. We don't know what they say when we can't hear.
Dakarai: You have to separate the person from the language. They find it very good that we [also] speak English with the children.... I try not to speak Afrikaans – not to identify myself with that language.

In the concluding chapter of the book we will consider support for trilingualism and threats to it from outside the family, at local, national and international level. Those threats include the attitudes of others, the impact of English as a global language and the uncertain future of some minority languages. We will also provide some examples of families who pursued trilingualism successfully, 'against the odds'.

Summary

Our plan is to cover the major issues that parents highlighted in research interviews, in their comments on the internet forum and in anonymous emails. We hope that by the end of the book readers will feel able to answer the major questions posed in this chapter about the strategies that can be employed at home and outside in order to foster particular languages with their children and about the influence exerted on the outcome by parents' own linguistic and cultural backgrounds, and by the beliefs and attitudes of members of the extended family, as well as people beyond the family. We will try to provide readers with suggestions and recommendations based on our own research and on the current literature, which is presented in the next chapter.

2 Comparing Bilingual and Trilingual Families

Introduction

The aim of this chapter is to introduce readers to some of the research that has been done in the fields of bilingualism and trilingualism. We have not attempted to provide an exhaustive account but instead have selected research that we think will be of particular interest and relevance to parents in trilingual families and their advisers. A list of references and further reading, which covers much of the research literature in the field, is provided at the end of this book. This chapter sets the scene for a better understanding of the chapters that deal with specific challenges and difficulties that trilingual families may face during their journey of raising multilingual children.

While the study of trilingualism is rather recent, bilingualism has been established as a research subject in its own right for over 100 years, attracting scholars in a variety of fields, such as linguistics, psychology and sociology. Many of the early studies were conducted by parents recording their own children's language development. For example, the influential idea of One Parent One Language was first described in print by Jules Ronjat in 1913, a French linguist married to a German speaker, who was living in Paris when their son, Louis, was born in 1908. Louis learned German from his mother and from his German nanny, while acquiring French from his father and from his contacts with French speakers in the area of Paris where they lived. Louis never confused the two languages and maintained a balance between them as he grew up. For example, it is reported that, while he preferred to read in German, he preferred to take his school examinations in French (see Ronjat, 1913). As we shall see, subsequent researchers, such as Barron-Hauwaert (2004), have continued to emphasise the value for bilingual learners of maintaining a balance between their two languages.

Much of the work on speakers of three languages has drawn on core ideas and theoretical concepts that were originally developed through research on bilingual speakers. But the development of trilingualism is much more complex than the development of bilingualism, and it is only relatively recently that researchers in linguistics and psychology have begun to study trilingual speakers. For example, in 2008 Xiao-lei

Wang reported on how her two sons came to learn three languages simultaneously. She had come from her native country, the People's Republic of China, to study at the University of Chicago, when she met her husband, who was an exchange student from the French-speaking part of Switzerland. Their sons, Léandre and Dominique, learned French (their father's language), Chinese (their mother's language) and English (the language of their parents' adopted country).

Using a framework that was designed to explain bilingualism as a way of organising our thinking about trilingualism may be misleading. A major reason for this is that three languages cannot be as balanced and equal as two languages. The risk of under-developing or under-using one, two or even all three languages is high. Perhaps children will use their mother's language very much more than their father's because they spend more time with their mother in their preschool years than with their father. We will demonstrate this in Chapter 4, through the example of a Bulgarian/Croatian/German family. The father, Drazen, worried a great deal that Croatian was not used often enough, because his Bulgarian wife, Bisera, spent most of the time with their six-month-old daughter. Drazen said:

> Bisera is together with the little one the whole day – so she doesn't need to worry as the child will learn Bulgarian as she is together with her all the time.... I am the one with a disadvantage because of my work and time I can spend with the little one. So we have conflicts as I have nightmares that I can't spend time with my daughter and as a result she won't learn Croatian properly, if at all. My worst scenario is that she starts talking to me in Bulgarian.

On the other hand, some parents may find that their children will use the main language of the society in which they live much more than the languages of either parent, because they have a local nanny or spend time in a local children's centre or nursery. In fact, we found in our research that, often, multilingual parents who had also spoken the community language from childhood dropped their second native language, because the children started to prefer the community language. Since this was also a native language for most Group 2 and Group 3 parents, they might then drop the minority language. For example, Ablerus, a Greek/British father whose situation is described in Chapter 4, had found it increasingly difficult to use Greek since the children started nursery. Ablerus said:

> Now the children will hear my voice and then I am beginning to hear them as well answering in Greek. It is a conscious decision and it is hard work, especially when they go to school and suddenly they speak a lot more English.

Despite the obvious differences and challenges, trilingualism has often been seen as another type of bilingualism simply because there is very little research available that specifically compares trilingual speakers or families with those who are monolingual or bilingual. However, while children who are learning three languages face most of the tasks that are associated with bilingualism, they have some unique and more

Table 2.1 Bilingual and trilingual acquisition orders

	Bilingual acquisition orders	*Trilingual acquisition orders*
1	First L1 then L2	Fist L1 then L2 then L3
2	First L2 then L1	First L1 then L3 then L2
3	L1 and L2 simultaneously	First L2 then L1 then L3
4		First L2 then L3 then L1
5		First L3 then L2 then L1
6		First L3 then L1 then L2
7		L1 and L2 simultaneously then L3
8		L1 and L3 simultaneously then L2
9		L2 and L3 simultaneously then L1
10		L1 and L2 and L3 simultaneously
11		First L1 then L2 and L3 simultaneously
12		First L2 then L1 and L3 simultaneously
13		First L3 then L1 and L2 simultaneously

Note: L1 = language 1; L2 = language 2; L3 = language 3.

challenging tasks in addition. So the process is likely to be different, as pointed out by Jasone Cenoz (2000) from the University of the Basque Country. For instance, when two languages are learned, there are only three possible orders for learning them: a child might learn, say, French first and then German; or German first and then French; or German and French simultaneously. But when three languages are acquired, there are 13 possible acquisition orders: there could be a simultaneous acquisition of all three languages, or one language might be acquired after the first one has been established, or two might be acquired simultaneously while the third one is learnt later (see Table 2.1).

We found that Group 1 families in our study (see Chapter 3) usually followed order 7 – L1 and L2 simultaneously and then L3. L1 and L2 are the parents' native languages and L3 is the community language. For example, Hanna, a Finnish mother, and Hans, a German father, used their respective native languages with their two children. English, the community language, was added when the children started nursery. On the other hand, Group 2 families (see Chapter 4) usually followed acquisition order 10, that is, using all three languages from the beginning, simultaneously. We will show in Chapter 4 that this can be a difficult undertaking, as bilingual parents tend to drop a minority language when the children become older and have their own language preferences. This was the case with Alberto, a US-American/Italian father, who found it difficult to use two languages with his children. Eventually the children wanted to speak only English with him. Alberto said: 'My daughter understands Italian very well, but then she says: "say it in English". And then I say it in English.' Edda, his Dutch wife, added: 'Being exposed is no burden; speaking is different, like telephoning the father when the children want to put down the receiver because they don't want to have stress with Italian.'

In giving these examples of language use, we need to be cautious with our assumptions, as these orders can and usually do change when trilingual families move to other communities or countries. In fact, this seems to be quite common, as many parents in our study commented that they had changed their place of residence a number of times. In these circumstances, language use changes dynamically as families adapt to the new language environments. This was also the case for Alberto and Edda, as described above, who had lived in Germany for seven years before moving to England in 2001. Very soon, the children preferred speaking English, while German became a minority language, which only the parents spoke, as a lingua franca. Even this seemed to change as English became ever more dominant in everyday situations. Edda said: 'It's more English as a common language.... Even if my husband tries to speak Italian, it often ends up with English.' As our case studies in later chapters will show, the interactions between what each parent speaks and what is spoken in the local community may be very complex. Thus a trilingual system is fundamentally different from a bilingual one, both for the individual and for the family. So when research into how children learn three languages is based exclusively on ideas from research into bilingualism, it may not ask the most important or most appropriate questions.

Do Children Who Are Learning More Than One Language Get Confused?

In spite of all those points of difference, however, we can still learn a great deal from bilingual studies. Even when a bilingual speaker uses two languages with the same level of knowledge and skill as native monolingual speakers, they do not function psychologically exactly like two monolinguals in one body. Philip Herdina and Ulrike Jessner noted in 2002 that multilingualism is not multi-monolingualism: it involves a different combination of language competencies. In contrast to monolinguals, multilinguals have a different knowledge of their first language, a different awareness of how language works and different systems for processing language. In the early 1980s, the Canadian linguist Jim Cummins proposed the 'iceberg analogy' to illustrate bilingualism in the brain. It was assumed that bilingual speakers' proficiency in both their languages is based on a shared underlying 'languages' system in the brain, where the underlying principles of linguistic knowledge are stored, such as a basic understanding of grammar and syntax. This suggested to Cummins that the learning of two or more languages might be supported by one shared processing system, especially when the languages are acquired in a balanced way (see Figure 2.1).

The iceberg analogy is a simplified illustration or model of how the acquisition of two languages might be supported in the brain. Linguistic and cognitive skills are

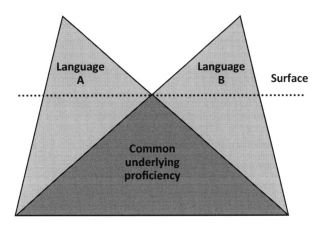

Figure 2.1 The iceberg analogy

interdependent because they draw on a common underlying proficiency. In the analogy, the two languages are joined together below the surface, but above the surface they are separate. There is empirical evidence that is consistent with this model. For example, it has consistently been found that, although young children often mix languages unsystematically at first, that usually fades if both languages are learned in a balanced way. This suggests that the two languages are not interfering with each other but instead complementing (and even stimulating) each other cognitively and linguistically.

There is a good deal of research supporting this model, such as from Jürgen M. Meisel in 1994 and 2011. He showed that even two-year-old bilingual children learning to speak French and German achieved correct verb placement in each language. This was evidence that young bilingual children can use the correct grammatical rules in each language and show an awareness of different communication contexts. In another study, published in 2002, Virginia C. Mueller Gathercole from Bangor University compared seven- and nine-year-old Spanish/English bilinguals with English monolinguals. She found that younger bilingual children did not learn the correct syntactic forms as well as monolinguals, but older bilinguals did equally well as monolinguals. This means older and more balanced bilinguals are more like monolinguals in terms of language competence.

When Cummins' model was introduced over 30 years ago, there had been little detailed research on the brain mechanisms underpinning bilingualism. Since then, new methods have been developed for studying the brain (see below), and this research has provided some support for Cummins' basic ideas. For example, a team led by Laura-Ann Petitto at the University of Toronto took a particular interest in the ability of young infants to discriminate the sounds of their language when they hear them, even before they begin to babble and make such sounds themselves. From soon after birth, babies are able to discriminate between phonetic units, the smallest 'building blocks' of language, from any of the world's languages. But early in their second year they lose the ability to do this for all sounds and, instead, hone in on the sounds that are heard most often in their native language with increased precision. Studies in Petitto's lab and elsewhere showed that babies who were exposed to two languages showed 'an increased sensitivity to a greater range of phonetic contrasts, and an extended developmental window of sensitivity for perceiving these phonetic contrasts relative to monolingual children' (Petitto, 2009: 5).

This work was followed up later by studying the brain activity of monolingual and bilingual infants during tasks that involved visual perception or speech recognition. The researchers used functional near infrared spectroscopy (fNIRS) to test what neural tissue networks were involved in linguistic perception tasks as against general perceptual processing tasks. (fNIRS is a non-invasive technology that allows the researcher to monitor blood flow in the brain.) They found that the brain's main language areas were employed in similar ways in very young bilingual and monolingual babies. They appeared to activate specific language-dedicated neural tissue for processing sounds that were associated with their languages in the same way that they activated the area of the brain associated with visual processing when they were looking at a non-linguistic visual checkerboard. Like the evidence on the development of phonetic perception, this appears to offer support for Cummins' original simple model of a common underlying proficiency that facilitates the learning of two languages. There is more general information later in this chapter on the blossoming research on bilingualism in the brain.

How far can all this evidence from the study of bilingual children apply to trilingual learners? The language situation for trilinguals is more complex than for bilinguals in terms of the psychological benefits. It is often assumed that trilingualism has a positive effect just like bilingualism, but unfortunately solid studies and tests are still missing. Balancing three languages is challenging and needs strong support from parents and the community. In fact, in our study, trilingual parents found it hard to use three languages and very often ended up using only one. Two recent completed doctoral studies on trilingual children have attempted to explain how children mix and switch their languages. Ksenija Corinna Ivir-Ashworth (2011) examined two trilingual children of the same family growing up with Croatian, English and German from birth. She found that even when they were young, the children showed sensitivity in their language switching by selecting the correct language for specific social situations. For example, they combined words and grammar from more than one language in order to communicate more effectively and with more complexity, but normally only when talking with someone who would understand both languages. Language mixing is often regarded as a deficiency but it may, rather, be a sign of the child's linguistic and social creativity.

Elena Davidiak (2010) also studied language switching, in two trilingual sisters aged six and nine. These children used their trilingual ability to include or exclude people from a conversation. Language mixing within sentences was more apparent in the younger sibling, but this was related not only to age but also to personality differences.

Davidiak emphasised that lexical need was only one of the causes for the two girls switching languages within a sentence. The other important factor for language switching was seen to be the social demands of the situation, such as when they were talking to different people who spoke different languages or when they wanted to indicate a change of a conversational subject. Similar observations have been made of children who are developing bilingually. In each case the detailed analysis of language switching has indicated the purposeful use of the child's full linguistic repertoire rather than an experience of confusion or uncertainty.

Does Learning More Than One Language Enhance Cognitive Growth?

From the early 19th century to about the 1960s, research into bilingualism seem to support the idea that bilingual children inevitably suffer from academic retardation and have a lower IQ than monolingual children. Over the last 50 years empirical studies in many different countries and with many different language combinations have shown that this is not the case. The earlier research had often been designed in a way that created a bias against bilingual children showing their thinking skills at their best. For example, the tests that were used would be presented in the bilingual learners' second language. When researchers developed unbiased testing procedures, the apparent cognitive limitations associated with bilingualism disappeared.

In fact, bilingual speakers enjoy a number of specific cognitive advantages that are not so easily available to those who are monolingual. One of the best established of these is the ability to think flexibly. This has been demonstrated in 12-month-old infants from bilingual homes even before they learn to speak. In 2009, Agnes Melinda Kovács and Jacques Mehler were working on a study in Trieste (Italy), where bilingualism has historic roots. In this research, half of the infants lived in homes where both parents spoke only Italian, and half had parents with different mother tongues, who addressed them in different languages on a daily basis. Many, for example, heard Italian and Slovenian, while others heard Italian and Spanish or French or English or Croatian. The children listened to simple speech sounds that had a different structure (e.g. *lo-lo-vu* and *lo-vu-lo*). Pictures of attractive toys were associated with these structures, and the researchers measured how quickly the infants learned to look in the place where they would find a toy after hearing a particular sound. When given the opportunity to simultaneously learn two different regular patterns of association of this kind, the bilingual infants learned both, whereas the monolinguals generally learned only one. Kovács and Mehler concluded that the bilinguals were more flexible learners.

In older children this flexibility has been shown in various forms, such as efficient selective attention. For example, they can ignore extraneous information in verbal tasks more effectively than monolingual children of the same age (probably because they get practice in doing so when they need to listen or speak in one language and suppress the use of their other language). This enhanced capacity for selective attention extends to tasks which do not involve language directly. One well established instance of this involves the use of picture cards, each of which has a circle or a square that is either red or blue. Children are asked to sort the cards initially by one dimension, for example colour. In 1999 Ellen Bialystok, working in Toronto, reported that groups of monolingual and bilingual children aged three to six years performed equally well on this task. But when the dimension was switched so that the cards had to be sorted by the other dimension (e.g. shape), the bilingual children handled the requirement to shift attention much more successfully than the monolingual group.

Advantages such as these are most likely to be found in older children and adults who are 'balanced' bilingual speakers, those who continue to develop their languages more or less equally. Often, though, one language is learned less well or used less often or used in less demanding contexts. The effect will be that one language comes to dominate the other, and that may lead to the under-development of the weaker language and even to its demise. The dynamic factors in this process are described in the 'threshold theory', which was developed by the Canadian linguist Jim Cummins in 1979. Its aim is to describe language competence and whether it has effects on bilinguals' awareness of how languages work, for instance the way in which grammatical rules that differ between languages may serve the same functional purpose in supporting effective communication (see Figure. 2.2).

The threshold theory refers to two thresholds. Children who do not pass the first threshold, 'limited bilinguals', usually learn a low-status minority language at home (L1) which they do not develop to a high level of competence before they are exposed

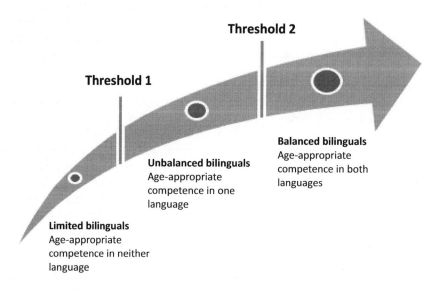

Figure 2.2 Threshold theory

to a higher-status majority language outside the home (L2) in preschool settings and eventually in school. They start learning L2 with a disadvantage and do not continue to develop L1 beyond a basic level. The impact on their intellectual development is negative: they bring weak linguistic resources to every cognitive task they face in school and outside. As a result they do worse, on average, than their monolingual peers in the school curriculum. Those who pass the first threshold become 'unbalanced bilinguals', with a level of competence in one of their languages that is appropriate to their age. For example, they may have sufficient competence in the majority language to function successfully in a classroom where it is the main medium of communication. Children in this group – those who have passed the first threshold – are likely to show neither positive nor negative effects on their cognitive development. Their performance on most cognitive tasks will be comparable to that of their monolingual peers. Those who pass the second threshold, 'balanced bilinguals', maintain their development of competence in L1 while building up their competence in L2. Their age-appropriate competence in both languages is likely to have positive cognitive advantages of the kind described above.

That picture of two thresholds and three levels of balanced or unbalanced competence across two languages can be applied to bilingual children fairly easily, and the research that has been done with them as a result has produced clear results. We can describe the conditions in which learning two languages enhances cognitive growth and those in which it does not. In the case of children learning three languages, the picture is inevitably more complex and there has been little research. We suspect that the family groupings described in Chapter 1 will prove to be useful in predicting whether trilingual children enjoy the benefits of enhanced cognitive growth. Perhaps the experience of children living in a Group 1 family will help them to do better than their monolingual peers in tests like Bialystok's card-sorting task. However, this research has not yet been attempted. Other ideas on how multilingual proficiency may influence development in different ways from bilingual proficiency will be explored later on in this chapter.

How Does the Development of the Brain Differ When a Child Becomes Bilingual?

In a 2009 report entitled 'New Discoveries from Bilingual Brains', Laura-Ann Petitto and Kevin Niall Dunbar, two neuroscientists from the University of Toronto, reviewed evidence comparing the brains of monolingual and bilingual children and adults. As noted above, much of the research had used the non-invasive brain imaging technique fNIRS (functional near-infrared spectroscopy) to monitor brain activity. During these experiments, as described above, monolingual and bilingual infants showed the same involvement of neural tissue in the brain dedicated to language, which suggested that young speakers of one language and speakers of two languages focus attention on their native language(s) in similar fashion. The two groups also had identical robust activations in the brain's classic language areas when they were processing phonetic sounds and words. As babies from monolingual and bilingual homes grew older, similar brain changes were observed with age, for example in relation to established language milestones such as babbling, talking in single syllables and forming complex sentences. Focusing on these language milestones, Kovelman and Petitto (2002) found that exposure to two languages before the age of five years was optimal for bilingual language development and dual language mastery. Experimental results even suggested that early bilingual exposure leads to a 'bilingual advantage' in phonetic processing. This means that babies from a bilingual home show an increased sensitivity to a greater range of phonetic contrasts than infants from a monolingual home.

Other studies, such as from Susan Perry, have reported similar results. For example, it appears that young bilinguals show much more activity in the language-dominant left hemisphere of the brain when they toggle between their languages. This has been called a 'neurological signature' for multilingualism, because the neural activity is so prominent and predictable on brain scans. It has been found most clearly in bilingual speakers who were proficient in both languages and learnt them before the age of five. There were more differences recorded between 'early exposed bilinguals' and 'late exposed bilinguals' (those who learned a second language as adults). Using brain imaging techniques during behavioural tasks, Laura-Ann Petitto and Kevin Niall Dunbar reported that 'early exposed' bilingual adults utilised the left hemisphere of their brain for each language in the same way that monolinguals do for theirs. But, when bilingual speakers who had learned a second language in adulthood were studied, the brain scan results suggested that key centres for their languages were located further apart from each other. The implication is that becoming bilingual later in life requires a different form of neural organisation for language processing from what is familiar from studying monolingual speakers, but becoming bilingual in childhood does not.

In summary, the evidence from neuroscience is strongly supportive of the efforts that some multilingual families make to introduce their children to more than one language early in life.

Does a Child's Place in the Family and School Affect Use of the Family's Languages?

Among the other important factors that influence the acquisition of bilingualism, one that is a concern to many parents is the impact of a child's place among the siblings in the family. In her book *Bilingual Siblings*, Suzanne Barron-Hauwaert (2011), who is a mother of bilingual children herself, examined this (among many other factors shown to be important). She studied her own family's language practices and reviewed other family research. Her three children seemed to face different challenges with their two languages, partly because they had friends who spoke different combinations of languages and partly because they had different approaches to language learning. For example, one child was more persistent in trying to make sure his language was always accurate, while the others were more concerned with getting their message across, even if language mixing was needed. In a survey she conducted of parents in bilingual families, Barron-Hauwaert found that most of the parents did not think that bilingualism was easier to maintain in one-child families. Although there might be more quality time with the child, sibling bonding and interaction were seen as more important.

Usually, younger siblings are guided by older ones in terms of language preferences, and this is often decided by the older siblings' increasing preference for the main language used in their formal education. In fact, there are many studies showing that the school language becomes the dominant language within bilingual contexts. For example, Barbara Zurer Pearson, who wrote the book *Raising a Bilingual Child* (2008) and many research articles, studied the language preferences of immigrant junior high school pupils in the USA. She found that, shortly after arriving in their new country, immigrant children began to show a preference for using English over their home language. A study reported in 2005 by Cathy Benson-Cohen, a mother of bilingual children, showed similar results in a bilingual family living in France, where the language of schooling also became the preferred language of siblings aged eight and nine years. The impact can be found even earlier, as shown in a study by Ludo Verhoeven and Hendrik Boeschoten in 1986, who examined the use of Turkish by children born to Turkish-speaking parents in the Netherlands and in Turkey. They found that the development of skills and knowledge in their home language began to stagnate from the age of four years in the group who attended Dutch kindergartens. Slowly, Dutch words and grammatical forms began to emerge in their use of Turkish. There are many anecdotal accounts of how these changes in the preferences of older siblings have a major impact on the language practices and preferences of their younger brothers and sisters.

This is a process that affects bilingual and trilingual families in the same way: the community language to which the children are exposed at school comes to dominate their lives. Xiao-lei Wang (2008) suggested that parents need gentle but firm determination if they are to resist these external social pressures. Writing about her trilingual children growing up in the USA with French, Chinese and English, she described a range of strategies that she, as a native Chinese speaker, and her husband, as a native French speaker, had employed during the children's crucial early kindergarten years. These included helping them to describe their school experience in the home languages, helping them to form the habit of asking when they did not know a word or expression in the home language, and matching school reading and writing in English with home reading and writing in the home languages.

Developing Ideas on How Multilingualism Differs from Bilingualism

Recent research on multilingualism has made it clear that those who learn three or more languages are in a qualitatively different position from bilingual learners. One model that illustrates this was developed by Philip Herdina and Ulrike Jessner (2002) – the 'dynamic model of multilingualism'. This suggests that as children acquire more than two languages, they come to notice similarities and differences between them and develop new skills through learning how languages work. It is expected that this will facilitate the learning of subsequent additional languages as they explore and make use of the basic mechanisms of languages. There are many routes and pathways to trilingual language development. We must therefore ask whether all the children will benefit in this way or whether the outcome may depend on the circumstances or the sequence of their exposure to their languages.

David Lasagabaster, working in the Basque country in the late 1990s, studied 252 students aged 10–14 years who were bilingual in Basque and Spanish and were learning English at school. His study was designed to determine how the threshold theory (described above) might need to be adapted in order to cover trilingual learners. He examined the students' performance on tests of 'metalinguistic awareness' (the understanding of how language principles operate across languages). The results showed no significant differences between those who were highly competent in three languages and those who were highly competent in only one or two languages. Later studies have suggested that the learning of a third language by children who have already acquired two languages at the same time in early childhood may follow a route that is similar to that followed when monolingual speakers learn a second language. Whether they have enhanced metalinguistic awareness or other cognitive advantages will depend on such factors as the age at which each language is learned, the balance between them and whether they have continuing opportunities to use all of them.

In 2004, Michael Clyne, Claudia Rossi Hunt and Tina Isaakidis of the University of Melbourne, Australia, reported on an investigation of the impact of learning a third language on 44 bilingual students in that city. The study focused on bilinguals learning another community language (Greek or Spanish) as a third language through specially designed secondary school language programmes. The study participants spoke a wide range of languages at home in addition to English (25 different languages, of which the most common were Filipino and Italian). Some of the findings suggest that the bilingual speakers tended to be more persistent and effective learners of the target language than monolinguals. They themselves suggested that this might be because they benefited from their enhanced metalinguistic awareness. They thought that through learning a third language, their maintenance of their home languages was strengthened, because they developed a more general interest in languages. Some of them reported that, as a result, they spoke their home language more often than before in public places. A number of them even expressed the desire to pursue the study of languages later on or mentioned the possible benefits of multilingualism in their future work in Melbourne, in communicating with people who cannot speak English, and in travelling and working overseas. We need to keep in mind that the study was conducted in Melbourne, a multilingual and multicultural environment where many people are aware of different traditions and languages. It is possible that this means that the findings will be less applicable to predominantly monolingual societies.

Summary

In this selective review of research on bilingualism and trilingualism we have concentrated on ideas and concepts that we expect to be of interest to parents in multilingual families. Trilingualism involves more than speaking three languages, as it requires a complex linguistic and cultural awareness which monolingual speakers do not normally have. The studies outlined in this chapter highlight some advantages that early bilinguals and multilinguals have over monolinguals linguistically and also cognitively. Recent brain research suggests that this may extend to fundamental neuropsychological benefits. Despite this, more research is needed to see how far findings from studies of bilingual speakers are equally true for trilingual speakers. Bilingualism and trilingualism are dynamic and change constantly, depending on age, siblings, work, friendships and school. In societies that are based on monolingual expectations, the benefits of bilingual and trilingual proficiency are sometimes very difficult to realise. In the next three chapters we will discuss how this impacts on different types of trilingual family.

3 Monolingual Parents Living Abroad (Group 1)

Introduction

In this chapter we discuss what we learned from parents in the first group of families. These are trilingual families in which each parent speaks one different native language while they live as a family in a country where the community language is added as a third language (they speak that language as an additional, non-native language). The parents have no common native language.

Figure 3.1 summarises the language background of Group 1 families (see also Figure 1.1, p. 5, for all three groups of trilingual families). We found that parents in this situation were particularly motivated to raise their children trilingually. Most of them used their native languages 'naturally' with their children inside and outside their

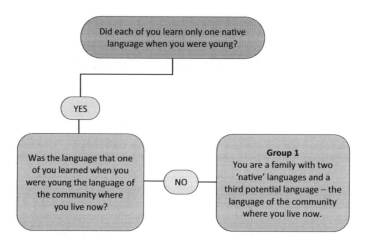

Figure 3.1 Language background tool – Group 1

homes, because it was their strongest and most familiar language. Ulivia, who grew up in Italy, said: 'I felt that the only language I could use with my daughter was Italian. I couldn't speak to her in English, it doesn't feel natural. I don't know why – it's just not my language.' In this chapter we will try to explain the language choices that this group of parents made with their children. We will look at:

- the ways they used their languages with their children;
- the effects that their proficiency in their languages had on their decision;
- the plans they made for their children's education and the effects those plans had once the children started school;
- the influence on them of the wishes of their extended families;
- their thinking about whether and how they would try to pass on the culture of their own childhood home to their children.

(a) The Parents' Strategies at Home

Many parents in this situation began working towards trilingual development even before their children started to talk. They employed the One Parent One Language (OPOL) strategy. Each parent used their own native language with the children so that they were exposed to two native languages at home. The parents did not use the community language at home, and so the children acquired that third language later, in nursery, school and the general community. In this group of families the parents could employ the OPOL strategy as an effective and workable means to raise their children trilingually. (For a discussion of the advantages and disadvantages of the strategy for other types of trilingual families see Chapters 4 and 5.) In addition, many families built networks with other trilingual or bilingual families, which created a supportive and appreciative environment for using the OPOL method.

Claire and Ken

Ken, who was 39 years old, came originally from Canada. He had been living in Germany for 13 years together with his wife, Claire, who was the same age and grew up in France. The parents spoke English with each other because the mother felt that she did not 'have a choice, as my husband barely spoke German and French even less. So there was only English possible.' Nonetheless, the parents had started to use more German with each other because it had improved since they came to Germany 13 years earlier. However, with their three children, aged 3, 8 and 10 years, they used only their respective native languages, English and French, inside and outside their home.
Claire said:

German wouldn't be natural for me but I don't mind French or English; it's not important as long as the children speak it properly and as long as they don't mix... I can't change it. I have to speak French and Ken can't speak anything else than English to the children. Somehow it's not an effort.

Claire's parents were Moroccan emigrants who came to 'France by force because of the war. For them it was important to integrate and forget that they came from there and suddenly the whole family became French.' Claire found it a 'pity' that her parents did not use their native languages with her and neither did the father's parents employ any of their home languages.

My parents are polyglots both. My mother is Portuguese brought up in Morocco. Also she can speak Portuguese and French. My father was born in Germany and has lived in Asia and Morocco.... They don't find multi-lingualism positive because they had problems as foreigners in France when they came from Morocco.

Claire added:

On my husband's side his parents were German. They immigrated to Canada and my father-in-law even forbad speaking German. Also with his wife they started to speak English and therefore the children did not learn German.

Most parents in this group showed similar patterns in the way in which they used their respective native languages with their children, because it came 'naturally' and without an 'effort'. They also believed that multilingualism benefits a person. Most parents had learnt the community language but they did not consider it a language to use with their children, because they felt that they were not capable of using it like a native speaker. Parents emphasised that having a high level of competence in their own languages allowed them to feel confident when they were speaking to their children. So their language practices were partly based on their sense of proficiency in their native languages. At the same time, the parents in this group regularly referred to their limited proficiency in the community language as a reason not to use it with their children. Brunilda, a Portuguese mother, said: 'We can't speak perfect German, which would not be nice if the children learnt broken German from us'.

As part of the research interviews, parents were also asked to reflect upon what they saw as positive and what they saw as negative in a child developing three languages. This group of parents highlighted positive aspects more than any other group. For example, Adrian, a Dutch father who was living in Germany together with his Brazilian wife, Gabriela, and their six- and eight-year-old children, said:

Our children can live with trilingualism very well. I don't see any negative points about it but it is easier now that they know three languages later on in school. And when they have to learn languages it's going to be easier for them; that's what I think anyway. And if our eight-year-old son goes somewhere travelling it's quite easier to find a language they know.

We also found that the lingua franca between the parents did not markedly influence their language choices with their children. Often, Group 1 parents could not speak each other's native language and therefore they used mainly English between themselves. To their children, however, they used their respective native languages as a 'natural reflex'.

Summary

Most of the parents who spoke only one native language employed the OPOL method as a workable strategy to raise their children trilingually. Group 1 had more parents bringing up their children to speak three languages successfully than did the Groups 2 and 3. This was partly related to the parents' proficiency in their native languages, but other factors also played a part. Those factors are discussed in the rest of this chapter.

(b) Languages at School: Exposure to the Community Language

How did school policies influence the parents' use of languages at home in this group? Because they did not speak the community language as one of their native languages, they appeared to have a problem. Most of the schools in England and Germany, which have traditionally been monolingual countries, relied entirely on the main national language in their delivery of the curriculum and their management of pupils. So the parents needed to find strategies in order to make the community language available to their children from a very young age. Their children had to speak the national (community) language in order to follow the lessons in school. At the same time, they often wanted the children to maintain and extend the other language competencies which they had begun to develop at home. With this in mind, some parents enrolled their children in multilingual schools or nurseries or part-time supplementary schools so as to support their home languages. In this section we will outline the different reasons parents in this group of families gave for choosing certain educational strategies in order to bring up their children trilingually.

Mary and Saladino

Mary and Saladino were the parents of a typical Group 1 trilingual family who described themselves as using three languages 'naturally'. Mary, the 45-year-old mother, who originally came from the USA, had been together with her Italian husband, Saladino, for 16 years. They had come to Germany six years earlier with the intention to move to another country in the future. Before that, the family had lived in Italy first, then in New York for two years and then in Italy again for four years. They had two children, aged 8 and 11 years, who were being brought up trilingually. The parents opted to use their respective native languages with each other and with their children, but without implementing the OPOL method: 'We switch languages constantly according to the context'.

The parents had opted to enrol their children in an international school to ensure their multilingual development. 'Our children attend the European School…, where they study in English and German. They have lessons once a week on Italian grammar.' According to Mary, their children had become so competent in English and German that they started to 'correct their father with his English and they correct their mother when she mispronounces German.' The family regularly visited their relatives in the USA and in Italy. 'When we go to America to visit my family, the other two languages are virtually forgotten during the visit.' The parents thought that using their native languages came 'naturally', without making a conscious decision. Mary said:

> I do not think of convenience as much as I do of language appropriateness…. It came naturally. We realised we probably would have bilingual children but we had no idea whatsoever that we would live in a third country when we married.

Some families in Group 1, unlike Mary and Saladino, did use the OPOL method, that is, each parent employed their own native languages with their children, while the community language was learnt mainly outside the house, in nurseries, schools and the wider community. The availability of the educational establishments seems to have given the parents the 'freedom' to use their native language without having to worry about their children's acquisition of the community language. Henricus, an Italian father, put it thus: 'Our son is fully immersed into an English environment at school, so [there is] no need to speak to him English at home'.

In some cases the parents' choice of schools for their children was influenced by their future plans, as some of them intended to move to another country, where the children had to be able to speak an additional language. For example, some parents in Germany chose multilingual education for the children so that they could develop English as well as German to an adequate level. This was augmented sometimes with basic work on other European languages too. Elle, an American mother, explained:

> Both children attend the European school…. My daughter is in the English section and the second main language is German. My son is in the Italian section and the second main language is English…. The children are very open-minded and non-judgemental when they come together with other children from other countries

and cultures. I think they feel like they belong to an exclusive club when they meet other children in similar situations to their own. Since my children attend the European school, we've had positive experiences being 'Internationals' here in Germany. The school environment caters to families such as our own.

A number of families in Germany took their children to international English schools, even though they were not native English speakers themselves. This meant that the children were actually acquiring English as a fourth language, through schooling. As Ken, a Canadian father, explained: 'The European school is fantastic: they are all integrated. They speak all languages with each other. It fits our life and situation.' (See Chapter 6 for more information on international schools.) Despite the strong support for multilingualism and the dominance of English in these schools, the community language seemed to remain the children's preferred language outside the classroom. Carl, a Swedish father, said: 'A lot of the kids are growing up here, so therefore they use German. When there is a break they still use German regardless of which section they are, in French, Italian or English.'

Some parents expressed a concern that if they used English as a non-native language in a multilingual context, it might interfere with their children's acquisition of their own native languages. However, English was an important language for many of the families living in Germany in this sample, as the parents often worked in an English-speaking environment and they spoke English with each other as a couple. Riitta, a Finnish mother living in Germany, commented: 'We speak English together as a couple because we learnt to know each other in English.'

Similar considerations were cited by many of the parents living in England who spoke only one native language. They regarded English listening, reading, speaking and writing skills as essential for their children. So they had sent their children to English-speaking playgroups, nurseries or mainstream schools to provide them with English in an academic environment, while the home languages were used only at home. The combination of the language dominance, prestige and status of the English language seemed to have influenced most parents in this group in England to send their children to mainstream community-language nurseries or schools.

Additionally, in England some families in Group 1 had preschool children who would not be due to start school for some time. However, even with young children, the parents usually wanted their children to acquire English in nurseries or playgroups, because they were not using it at home. When Adriana and Frank, a Spanish/German couple in England, were asked how they provided their children with a trilingual environment, they answered:

We try to provide a trilingual one by means of speaking in Spanish and German and the third language comes here in England, because we have to communicate with each other and our son has to go to nursery and childminder.

Other families had tried to send their children to supplementary schools where they could learn the parents' native languages academically. But they often gave up because of the extra work. One example was Erum, an Iranian mother, who said: 'Actually we started this year in the beginning of schooling – we sent our son to a Farsi school but then we stopped. He had too much homework to do already, so we had to stop.'

Garret and Abbon, a Dutch/French couple who were living in England, had sent their children to a bilingual French/English school, but in the mother's opinion it created a gap between the children's acquisition of the home languages and the community language:

> Our children's Dutch is not as good as their French because they have never been in school. I think it would have been better to be in an English school because their English would have been perfect by now. I suppose, after three years in the European school, it's not the case.

There is a good deal of evidence that, when children start attending a local school, it can negatively affect their attitude towards their parents' native languages if those languages are not supported in the school. As a result, parents report that the language spoken in the nursery or school usually becomes the child's first language, putting the home languages in a detrimental position. Carl, a Swedish father, said: 'English was increasing as our son started now to prefer to use more and more English'. However, Carl and his Finnish wife, Emma, were determined to 'continuously' use their 'own languages', as were most of the other Group 1 families in our study.

Summary

As a strategy, most children Group 1 families learned their parents' native languages at home, while the community language was acquired in the neighbourhood, nurseries or schools. This released the parents to concentrate on their home languages, in which they felt more competent. This created a 'natural' language environment. Consequently, most of these children became very confident speakers of three languages. Sometimes the children even corrected their parents when they made mistakes in the community language or the language of the other parent. Most parents used the OPOL method. They switched languages only when the social context required it. Many of the parents who were living in Germany chose to send their children to multilingual schools, which usually supported English as a global language. They regarded multilingual education as a benefit for their children, as they could develop the community language and English at the same time to an adequate level.

(c) The Importance of the Extended Family

This section looks at the influence of the extended family on parents' language use with their children. As indicated above, the Group 1 families were very motivated to employ their home languages on a regular basis. So how was the distinctive language behaviour of Group 1 parents influenced by grandparents and other members of the extended family? We found that many of the parents used their native languages with their children partly because the grandparents could not speak the community language where the children lived. In order to communicate with their grandparents, the children needed to acquire the home languages that the older generation spoke, so as to have a 'communicative bridge'. Although other relatives and friends were mentioned too, they did not seem to be as influential. English, in particular, was so widely spoken that the children could use it with their cousins and friends. Galena, a Spanish mother whose husband, Erik, was Swedish, said: 'But again, the Swedish friends we have – they have children who are bilingual and so when they come here they [would] rather speak in English than Swedish'.

Brunilda and Patrick

Patrick, a 34-year-old Irish father who had been living in Germany for 12 years, was married to Brunilda, a 31-year-old woman from Portugal who worked as a skilled professional. Since the parents had married 10 years earlier, they had been living in Germany with the intention to stay. They had two boys, aged two years and one year, who were being brought up trilingually, learning English and Portuguese at home and German elsewhere. The parents decided to use English between them, the father's native language, because initially the mother's German was not so good and they had met in an English-speaking environment. According to the mother, her husband spoke only 'a bit' of Portuguese. When Brunilda was asked why the parents used their native languages with their children, she answered:

> For both of us the same reason. None of our parents speak a foreign language and we want our children to be able to communicate with their grandparents…. I think our children will learn German from friends, neighbours and in kindergarten.

Later in the interview, Brunilda again referred to the grandparents' inability to speak German as a major reason for their use of their native languages with the children at home:

> the grandparents want to communicate with their children. If I had different options like living in Portugal with a Portuguese husband, I would not care about three languages, but we have to use three languages also for the grandparents.

The parents felt that their children spoke German at a lower level than their peers. The older son in particular had initial problems in keeping the languages separate. Brunilda thought that acquiring multiple languages was a 'burden' for their older son, Mike, and 'perhaps he was confused, as he had only heard

> Portuguese from me and in the evening English from his father'. The mother also mentioned that, in general, the neighbours and other people in the community were 'very positive about trilingualism, at least in the town where we live. Our neighbours like it and so do our parents as they want to communicate with their grandchildren.'

Other parents Group 1 similarly referred to the grandparents and other relatives, who usually could not speak the community language of the country (England or Germany) where the families lived. Some of the parents made it clear that their main reason for using their native languages with their children was to provide a communicative bridge between their children and the relatives. 'It's simply so that our children could communicate with their relatives when they go back.'

Like Brunilda and Patrick, parents in this group used their respective native languages with their children partly because they thought that they did not speak the community language well enough and partly because the children's grandparents could not speak the community language at all. Some other parents also reported that, like Mike, their younger children did not speak the community language as fluently as local children. However, this did not deter the parents from using their native languages, as they gave priority to their desire for their 'children to be able to communicate with their grandparents'.

Summary

Some of the parents commented that their relatives were 'astounded' or 'amazed' that the children could speak three languages. For example, Gabriela, a Brazilian mother living in Germany, said: 'Most of them are amazed, like my parents if they hear the children speaking Portuguese'. This motivated the parents even more to use their native languages with their children. When the children got older, however, the community language became more dominant, partly because of the increase in vocabulary stimulated at school and partly too, it seemed, because of the influence of the peer group. Consequently, the home languages often developed into a simple communicative language with a rather basic vocabulary, which was enough to use for talking to the grandparents but had limited value in their lives otherwise.

(d) Cultural Practices and Language Use

The use of language is, in part, an expression of cultural identity. It is closely related to other aspects of a society's culture, including its traditions, values and customs. This part of the chapter examines the language practices of the parents in relation to their self-reported cultural background. Despite the fact that these families were faced with linguistic and educational challenges, they tended to be persistent in tackling the barriers against language maintenance. Cultural life added another component to the trilingual environment in which they lived. In this section we aim to identify the cultural factors that influenced parents' use of languages with their children. To what extent did the parents identify with the cultural background of their youth, and what impact did that have on their use of their native languages with their children?

Adriana and Frank

Adriana and Frank had been living in England for five years. Adriana had grown up in Spain and spoke Spanish as her native language, while Frank came from Germany and spoke German as his native language. Both parents also spoke English as a non-native language. Adriana was employed as a scientist, while Frank had recently started to work as a businessman. In the short term, they intended to stay in England, but they also had in mind to move to a 'German-speaking country, say Switzerland or Germany, because job-wise it would be easier, so we can have only two languages'. They had one 18-month-old son, who was being brought up trilingually, speaking German and Spanish at home and English in the nursery and with the childminder. When the parents were asked about the reasons for their language choices, they answered as follows:

Adriana: Well, for me it's extremely important that my son Anton understands and speaks Spanish because it's part of my identity and I want him to be part of that identity too.

Frank: Exactly, yes. Yes. I think I don't have anything to add. It's part of my identity, where I come from. In order to understand who I am, you need to understand the language as well.

Initially, the parents had spoken either Spanish or German with each other, but over time they had changed to using mainly English as the lingua franca between them. However, with their son, Anton, they continued using their respective native languages. English was seen as 'an additive' because they lived in England, where Anton was exposed to the language naturally. Adriana was worried by the idea that her son was going to be English:

I don't know, I have problems with the idea that Anton is going to be English. You see, I wouldn't mind him feeling German or feeling Spanish but if he feels English, I, personally, I would have to admit that it would be difficult for me because it's an alien country for me.

Moreover, the mother felt that her own and her husband's native cultural values were similar in some respects: 'We are very serious people and I think we are more German than you [Frank] are'. Frank agreed, saying that his wife's family was 'extremely organised, extremely efficient and correct'. Adriana related herself to German cultural values, despite the fact that she had been living in England for six years:

> I think I have been here for six years and I think that English people are very polite people, very nice, but I can't see that this is better for me at all. They express themselves in different ways, they have different values. So, six years is a long time and yet I feel closer to the German culture than to the English culture.

In the Group 1 families, each of the parents had a separate native language and neither spoke the local community language (English or German) as a native language. When we compared this group of families with other potentially trilingual families in this study, we found that most of these parents associated their native languages with their respective cultural background. 'Well, what I am, I am Greek'. This group of parents had grown up with one native language, in societies which usually had one main language, embedded in distinctive cultural traditions and historical and national values. Thus Elle, who had grown up in the USA and was married to Abramo, who had grown up in Italy, said:

> For me, speaking English keeps alive my Manhattan, the beaches of Florida, the Grand Canyon, Hollywood, the great vastness of America…. For my husband, speaking his language goes together with having a long delicious meal of pasta, speaking of politics, his Siena and Florence, corruption, chaos, artistic excellence, opera, the Pope…. Language and cultural identity for us just belong together.

Once the parents in this group had moved to a third country, a new culture and language were at their disposal, which had consequences for their children too. When we asked Abdera, who was from Greece, and Klervie, her husband, who was from France, about their language choices, they said:

Abdera: I think it was not a choice, it just happened like this. It happened that I am Greek and he [Klervie] is French, so we had the two languages. We take it as a matter of fact… it is our situation. I don't give up my language.
Klervie: Because our idea is that language is a culture, so we don't want the children to lose it, partly for themselves and partly for ourselves.

In this study, most parents regarded it as important that their children learn some of their native cultural values or that they feel in some way related to their cultural background. Claire, a French mother, said: 'It's important that I pass on my culture to the children, the French culture'. When parents in this group were describing their native cultural values, they generally referred to the following markers: language, family values, food, religious ceremonies or clothing. Language played an important part in their image of the culture of their childhood.

It is often suggested that in order to experience those cultural traditions at first hand it is necessary to travel to the home country. Some parents mentioned that they regularly visited their home countries to expose their children to the culture and language in a natural setting. Caela, who was from Croatia and was married to a man from Denmark, elaborated on this issue:

> In terms of home culture the main thing is that our children go once or twice either with us or alone to spend some time in Denmark or Croatia. And I hope they will be able to go to some kind of summer school or something like that so that they continue to have a kind of cultural expansion…. If our children do go back to Croatia or Denmark they can also integrate with other children and to have something in common, so they are not completely out of what is going on, because they can speak the language.

Summary

The fact that so many parents in Group 1 wished to pass on their native cultural values, traditions and customs to their children may have been a factor in their high success rate in bringing up their children trilingually. 'Of course I would like my daughter to learn about our cultural values. I think language is half of the culture.' Parents in this group tended to present a confident picture of their own cultural background, which they associated with their use of their native languages with their children. They had mostly grown up in societies which had one dominant language and cultural tradition. 'Our idea is that language is a culture.' Most of these parents wanted their children to learn about their native cultural values and customs, which also included the language as a cultural marker. 'I think if you take out the language out of the country then it is a bit difficult to bring the culture with it.'

Conclusion

In this chapter we have looked at factors that influence the language practices of families in which each of the parents had a separate native language and neither spoke the local community language (English or German) as a native language. These parents were particularly motivated to raise their children trilingually. Most of them used their native language 'naturally' with their children inside and outside their homes because it was their strongest and most familiar language. The specific language constellation within this group of families allowed the parents to use the OPOL method as an effective and workable strategy to raise their children trilingually.

As a strategy, most Group 1 parents spoke their heritage languages with their children, rather than the community language, which was a non-native language for this group of parents. As a result, the children needed community language support, which they received from local nurseries, schools and the general community in which they lived. Some families in Germany enrolled their children in multilingual schools so that their children could learn English in an academic environment.

Of similar importance was the influence of relatives, in particular the grandparents, on trilingual families' language practices. We found that approximately half of all the parents Group 1 had their relatives in mind when they decided to use their native languages with their children. These parents employed their native languages with their children partly in order to enable them to communicate with their grandparents and other relatives, who generally did not live in England or Germany and did not speak the language of the community where the parents resided.

And lastly, we examined whether the cultural background of the families in this group affected their language practices. These parents often referred to their original cultural background, native cultural traditions and values, which most of them wanted to pass on to their children. We also found that the majority of the parents in this group associated parts of their native cultural traditions and customs with their linguistic inheritance. This group of parents had mostly grown up in societies which had one dominant cultural tradition and one national language. They were committed to passing on parts of their native cultural values, customs and traditions to their children, which also included the language as a cultural marker. So the cultural backgrounds of the parents played a considerable role in their language choices with their children, in combination with their educational strategies, their language competence and the influence of relatives.

Implications for Parents (Group 1)

We found that parents in Group 1 were well placed to use the OPOL method as a strategy to maintain three languages. These parents each speak a different native language, which is not the main language of the community where they now live. In these circumstances it is helpful if each parent is as consistent as possible in using their respective native language with their children. For example, Baila, a Spanish-speaking mother, only used Spanish with her children, while the Finnish father spoke only Finnish to them. English was the language of the community. Parents have reported that this works well when the children are young. However, when the children start school or nursery it becomes harder to maintain the OPOL system because children spend a lot of time away from their parents, where they mostly speak the community language. In our research we also found that fathers seemed to struggle more than mothers with maintaining a heritage language, because they often worked long hours away from home. It may be helpful for a busy father to spend quality time in the evening, for example to read a storybook with his children or to play games in his heritage language (e.g. a game where children have to guess selected words or a board game published in his home country). An additional pressure is that most parents need to help their children with homework, for which they must use the community language of the school rather than a minority language. This is a true dilemma and challenge needing additional strategies. One suggestion is to temporarily use the community language during homework for example, but retain OPOL during other times.

It may be necessary to limit formal native language teaching with older children to one or two days per week, but it is important that parents use their native language with their children when they are young as much as possible, because this helps them develop a mental receptivity to multiple languages. Chapter 2 gives more detail about this process. It is necessary to strike a balance. On the one hand, parents require some determination to maintain the use of minority languages in the face of increasing pressure on the children to use the community language. On the other hand, parents will wish to ensure that the children associate their home languages with enjoyment and fun. That balance is easier to achieve when children are young. If a culture of minority language use is established at that stage, the children are more likely to find it natural to continue with it as they grow older.

If it is possible for families to travel to the parents' home countries regularly, that exposes the children to a natural language environment. They see their minority language in the context of the culture where others use it all the time. If they come to identify more with the associated culture, that will strengthen their motivation to use their minority language at home. It is especially valuable to create bridging experiences. If children are used to talking with their cousins or grandparents in the language of their parents' home country, it can be natural to continue using that language during occasional Skype or telephone conversations after they come home. If they become absorbed in a TV series or a local football competition while there, it will meet a felt need to follow that up once they are home. All such 'bridges' strengthen the link with the language and culture of the country of origin. Often, in addition, there are local relatives of Group 1 families, especially grandparents, who speak only one language, which will stimulate the trilingual child to practise the use of the minority language. Even young trilingual children are very good at detecting what language they need to speak in order to get their message across.

As trilingual children move into their teenage years, the maintenance of the minority languages becomes even more challenging. Parents' linguistic influence on their children diminishes, as in other areas of life. Teenagers pursue their own life and language preferences, and very often treat their peers as a reference group. That can lead them to give priority to the community language. As described in this chapter, Group 1 families were relatively successful in bringing up their children to speak three languages. We found that although trilingual teenagers may answer their parents in the community language, parents often continue to use their minority language. In this way teenagers continue to acquire the minority language in a receptive manner. This is the stage where the commitment during the earlier years of childhood pays off, because a basic knowledge of the language is fixed in the mind, even if some teenage trilinguals do not make much active use of it. The advice to parents is – continue to use your native language and be proud of it, even if your teenage child answers in the community language – they often understand more than they admit. We have given additional supportive ideas for trilingual families in Chapter 7.

4 One or Both Parents Are Bilingual (Group 2)

Introduction

In this chapter we will talk about trilingual families in Group 2, that is, families in which one or both of the parents speak two native languages (see Figure 4.1). This can include families where one parent speaks one native language and the other one two native languages. One of them may speak as a native language the local community language of the country where they now live.

Trilingual families in this group can also include families with parents who are both bilingual with the same language background but do not speak the local community language as a native language. There are other language backgrounds within this group but they are rare and will be covered only briefly (see Figure 1.1, p. 5, for a detailed

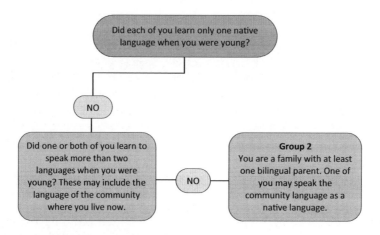

Figure 4.1 Language background tool – Group 2

illustration of all three main groups). We discovered from the survey interviews that many parents in this group dropped one of their native languages or were struggling with family trilingualism. This chapter provides an overview of trilingual families in Group 2 and how they were dealing with three potential languages. We will try to answer the following questions:

- In what ways do parents' language competencies influence their language choices with their children?
- How does the linguistic milieu in nurseries, schools and other communal establishments affect parents' language use with their children?
- What influence do grandparents and other relatives have on the parents' language decisions?
- In what ways do the cultural backgrounds of parents affect their language use with their children?

(a) The Struggle With Trilingualism

Family trilingualism does not come easily, especially in countries which are historically mainly monolingual. There are perceptions of how well children should speak, with an emphasis on native-like proficiency, especially for the community language. In Group 2 families, at least one parent was bilingual, which meant that they could not use the One Parent One Language (OPOL) method. Consequently, they found it a struggle to maintain one of their additional native languages. There were many possible reasons for this, such as the age of the children or the parents' language competence. Or they found it simply too much effort to use three languages at home. The following example describes a typical Group 2 family and how they were dealing with the challenges of trilingualism.

Tamara and Alex

Tamara, a 36-year-old German/Russian mother, was married to Alex, her 40-year-old German/Russian husband. This was a family where both parents spoke two native languages and had the same linguistic and cultural background. They both spoke Low-Saxon and Russian, while German had been acquired when they emigrated from the former Soviet Union to Germany 15 years earlier. The origin of 'Low-Saxon' (also called 'Low German') dates back to the 18th and early 19th centuries, when large numbers of German settlers came to Russia. These communities maintained a dialect of German that varied with their place of settlement in Russia and the area of origin in Germany. Most of the Germans, including many Mennonites, who settled in the Black Sea area, spoke Low-Saxon or Low-German (*Plautdietsch*, where *plaut* means 'flat' or 'low'). There are thus various groups of Low-German which resemble each other grammatically and lexically. For example, a speaker of Mecklenburg Low-German would be able to understand Low-German spoken by German/Russian immigrants from the Black Sea area of today's Ukraine. With the breakdown of the former Soviet Union, many of these German Russians migrated to America or returned to Germany, as was the case with Alex and Tamara. They brought Low-Saxon with them but found, of course, that, as in the former Soviet Union, it was not spoken outside their unique community.

Alex was employed as a manual worker, while Tamara stayed at home to look after their four children, aged eight, six and four years, and four months, who were all being brought up bilingually with Low-Saxon and German. When Tamara was asked why she had dropped Russian she said: 'We have thought simply about the children and for us as well. In Russia using Russian would have been an option but not in Germany, where we intend to stay. We would rather have English as a third language than Russian.'

The parents sometimes spoke Russian with their parents, who had also migrated to Germany, and when they did not want their children to understand. The grandparents spoke Low-Saxon, Russian and German to a reasonable level of competence. The family used Low-Saxon so that 'the children can cope with us as parents in the family and that the culture is not lost from our grandparents'. In fact, there was a big German/Low-Saxon community in the area, including a local church at which German/Low-Saxon and Russian were spoken, which had helped to preserve the Low-Saxon language and some of their cultural traditions as well. Tamara said: 'I would like that our children keep the Low-Saxon language, also that the culture is not lost and that they cope in the community surrounding'.

In addition, Tamara felt that her German was not so good because she had 'not learnt it properly', whereas both parents had learned Low-Saxon as their first language. They felt that they were 'more fluent and quicker' and they could 'express their thoughts better' in Low-Saxon. There was also a cultural component attached to their language choice, as Tamara pointed out:

> Low-Saxon is more something without a homeland [Heimat] and the culture is carried to Germany from that time. The Low-Saxon-speaking peoples have taken some cultural habits from Russia and the Ukraine. Now we are here but we are not really Germans but German Russians. But culturally we are more Low-Saxon and in Russia it was simply German culture. It's a mix.

This vignette tells a story that is typical of many of the Group 2 families who were interviewed. Bilingual parents tended to neglect one of their native languages, for various reasons. Some of them were worried that three languages would be too much for their children, while others were planning to introduce their children to an additional native language later, in order to establish confidence in two languages first. Palloma, a Spanish/French-speaking mother living in England, queried: 'My question in my mind: Is it better to introduce French when our son is two or three or four years, because it's an explosion of languages now he is saying a lot of words. Wouldn't it be a little bit too shocking for him?'

Raising children trilingually in predominantly monolingual societies requires a deliberate language maintenance strategy. One of the strategies that is discussed most frequently is the OPOL method. It requires each parent to use his or her native language consistently in order to avoid confusing the children. It is intended to enable the children to develop and then to maintain both their parents' native languages. The OPOL method was first used in bilingual families and many studies describe this method as a workable strategy to ensure a balanced usage of two languages (as Claire and Ken did, as described in Chapter 3). Each parent speaks just one language with the child, without mixing languages. Research studies have shown the advantages of OPOL, which makes it easy for children to recognise when they should speak which language to which parent. This enables the children to hold on to their parents' native languages.

Trilingual families are also beginning to experiment with the OPOL. However, there is an inherent instability and weakness in this method when three or more languages are involved. Using the OPOL for bilingual or trilingual parents means that they have to drop one or even two of their native languages. Which language is dropped may be determined by various factors, including language status, practicality or language competence. For example, it is rare for multilinguals to be equally competent in all language skills, reading and writing as well as listening and speaking in any one particular language; in addtion, usually one language is more dominant than the other. In most cases, multilinguals speak their different languages in different contexts, such as at home, at work or in school. Where and for how long each language is used can influence the competence in it. Multilinguals may find it difficult to interpret or translate, because they may not have an equivalent vocabulary in all their languages. It is also possible that a multilingual speaker may not feel confident in all the languages. Considerations of this kind may lead parents to decide to use an OPOL strategy, which means that the potential for trilingual development in the family is sacrificed.

We found that many bilingual parents did not speak their additional native language competently any more. This was a very common reason for parents Group to pull back from using all their languages with their children. Drazen, a Croatian father living in Germany, said:

> I must say I can express myself much better in German. I can't speak Croatian so well any more; it's just mixed. In the future I want to learn Croatian more intensively, not a course but with literature to bring back my Croatian as it once might have been. It doesn't help my daughter if I can't speak Croatian well so that she learns my mistakes. I need to speak it perfectly.

Summary

Many bilingual parents reported an imbalance between their two native languages, because one of the languages had not been used regularly since they came to England or Germany. This led most parents Group 2 to drop that language. Other researchers in the field of multilingualism have reported similar findings – that balanced trilingualism is difficult to achieve, because one or more languages are often at risk of becoming under-used. Some bilingual parents also commented that they found it impractical to use both languages unless educational support was given, which is explored in the next section.

(b) Education: Resignation or Challenge?

The parents Group 2 were in a position to pass on three native languages to their children between home and the community. Once the children were old enough to go to nurseries or schools, the parents could not spend so much time with their children. Therefore, language issues became a more prominent factor in the choices these bilingual parents made about schooling, because, for most of these families, the native language input at home was less than the community language input at school and in the neighbourhood. At this point, some parents in this group just surrendered to the overwhelming exposure to the community language, by dropping their native languages at home. Other parents used a variety of strategies to ensure that the children continued to develop trilingually, in spite of the obstacles. In this section we will look at the way in which some Group 2 families tried to maintain the three available languages in their families by making the influence of their children's nurseries or schools a positive one that supported that objective.

Telek

One father, Telek, was a second-generation 54-year-old Polish/British national who lived in England. His German wife had sadly died recently. When she was still alive, she used to speak English with her husband and German with their 14- and 17-year-old daughters, Karen and Sue. Telek started with Polish, but stopped doing so when the children started school. 'Sometimes if you wanted to speak Polish with the children they would refuse because all their friends were using English. This began since they started going to school, age of four to five.'

In this case, the children refused to speak Polish, as they had so many English-speaking friends from school. Moreover, the father had English as one of his native languages, so that the children may have questioned the need for additional languages, since they could communicate in English on a native level.

In the end, the father found it 'just easier to speak English', rather than push himself to use Polish.

> When the children were born I used Polish with the children. It came naturally, it just happened, and we thought we would continue because it felt good. But now it's English because all … anything meaningful now to the children is in English.

In addition, Karen and Sue had developed a native command of the German language, which was very helpful when they visited relatives in Germany. According to a friend of the family who was present at the interview, 'Karen and Sue speak German very well'. The mother had used German with the children when she was alive and they had learned German in school. In addition, the children spent time in Germany with their cousins. According to the father, his children did not have problems in Germany, because they could speak German fluently. The father also mentioned that his children had an initial language delay, which could have influenced his decision to be careful with multilingual language use. Nevertheless, the father felt that his children's English was now 'as good as their peers' if not better on occasions'. The family did not have much contact with Telek's relatives in Poland. Telek said that the children did not like going to Poland and that 'they haven't been to Poland on holiday but they like going to Germany. Yeah.'

We found that most bilingual parents in Group 2 dropped one of their available native languages. Those bilingual parents who were using both their languages with their children at the time of the survey had children who were still in their preschool years or who had only just started nursery or school. Bilingual parents found it easier to use their additional native language when their young children were still at home. However, with the beginning of mainstream preschool or nursery, maintenance of the home language became more difficult. Anastasia, a Cypriot/South African mother living in Germany described her experience of the issue: 'Hanna, my daughter, used to speak all three languages pretty okay before she started kindergarten. After that, life is not the same.'

The beginning of nursery and school marked an important milestone in these families' language practices, in that the parents had much less time with their children and, further, felt their children might be overwhelmed by new vocabulary taught in schools. Once the children became accustomed to their schools and the language that was spoken there, the bilingual parent in each of these families tended to discontinue the additional native language. Tanja, a Russian/English mother living in England, said: 'When my daughter was a baby, you see, I cuddled her and was speaking Russian to her and all that. Maybe all this started with English, maybe since she was two, maybe she was already in the nursery.'

Tiina and Ablerus

Ablerus, a 34-year-old father, grew up in England as a second-generation child of Greek immigrants. He was a fluent bilingual speaker of English and Greek, and his 32-year-old wife, Tiina, spoke Finnish as her native language. They had two sons, aged five and two and a half years, and a five-month-old daughter; the children were being brought up speaking Finnish and Greek at home and English in nursery, school and the wider community. It had become harder for the father to use Greek when his older son started school, because he only spoke English there. Ablerus said:

The issue was raised when our older son started school and he started speaking more English. I really had to work harder to speak Greek and you [his wife] were telling me to do so as well because it was to me so natural to answer in English. When they started going to school, especially the older one, I started speaking a lot more English to him.

At the same time, Ablerus was seeking other Greek-speaking people or places to support the use of Greek with his children: 'It really does help to go to the church or go to social events where they speak Greek'. The issue did not arise for Tiina, as English was a non-native language for her. Therefore, she spoke only Finnish with her children, who also generally spoke Finnish with each other. However, recently the children had started to use more English with each other because they were using it in playgroup and nursery. Tiina said:

I have to say, sometimes when Andrew, my older son, plays, like, car games, he does use English. And that started in nursery. When he went to nursery Andrew started to play in English. And now I have heard Franc, my younger son, who started playgroup a month ago, and I have heard him playing in English, which sounds weird because before that he never played in English, only in Finnish.

Some parents went to great lengths to find language support to maintain trilingualism in their family. For example, Palloma and Sam, who were currently living in a small town in England, were exploring the possibility of moving to a metropolitan area where French, one of Palloma's native languages, was supported through an international school. 'There is no French nursery here, so we are looking to move to an area where they have bilingual English/French.' There were other Group 2 families who had sent or were planning to send their children to multilingual schools, supplementary schools or multilingual nurseries to support their language development.

Some studies have shown that besides its linguistic advantages, multilingual education also benefits students' overall cognitive development and ideas (see

Chapter 2). Nonetheless, a number of people in the general public still have anxieties about bilingualism and even more about trilingualism. They tend to think of bilingualism as two language balloons inside the head. The monolingual has one well filled balloon, whereas the bilingual has two less filled or half-filled balloons. From the early 19th century till the 1960s, educational researchers commonly believed that bilingualism had a detrimental effect on children's intelligence. However, more recent studies using more advanced techniques have shown that bilinguals score higher on tests of verbal and non-verbal intelligence, although the answer to the 'cause and effect' question is not yet clear. More recent empirical studies in many different countries and with different languages have confirmed various aspects of the cognitive advantages in multilinguals. In particular, bilingual and multilingual education has been found to benefit students' overall cognitive and linguistic development, as they learn to move between languages in expressing complex thoughts and ideas. But more research is vital to give parents assurance that their children's trilingual upbringing is worth pursuing.

We found that many parents in Germany sent their children to bilingual German/English schools, sometimes because English was the native language of one of the parents, sometimes because of the status of English as a global language and sometimes for a combination of motives. Hailey, an American/Italian mother, commented on her German husband's use of English. 'My husband likes to speak English. It's not an effort for him and he uses English a lot in his job. So we just naturally speak English with each other even though we live in Germany.'

Sometimes multilingual schools created conflict between couples, because many parents who spoke a minority language did not find support outside their home, as bilingual schools usually supported English. One of these parents was Alin, a Romanian father who was living in Germany. He became anxious that his children would not develop fluent Romanian because the nursery supported only English, his wife's native language. In addition, the parents spoke English with each other, which meant that the only person speaking Romanian to the children was Alin. He said:

> It's difficult for me with Romanian because I am basically the only person who supports that language. It's obviously not difficult with English from my wife, as she does have a lot of support from friends, TV, in school and play groups, everything. Both my children go to playgroups and the activities are both in German and English. You start to wonder if it's really worth it if you are doing the right thing; like in my case, I am alone.

Summary

Some bilingual parents decided not to use their additional language even before their first child was born, partly because they felt these languages were not so useful. When we asked Hailey, an American/Italian mother, why she dropped Italian she said: 'Just because our children have really no reason to speak Italian in Germany.' Indeed, the majority of bilingual parentsGroup 2 stopped trying to use one of their native languages, either because they did not regard this language as useful or because the influence of school or nursery made it so difficult that they simply gave up. Once the children were older and had established themselves in school, they expressed their own language preferences. The bilingual parents who did try to use both languages mostly had preschool children. But as soon as the children started school or even nursery, this group of parents began to find it a struggle to maintain the use of one of their minority languages. Some couples tried to find strategies that would help them maintain trilingualism, such as sending their children to multilingual or supplementary schools or nurseries. Unfortunately, such schools were not always available and, when families did have access to such a school, they usually found that only the major European languages were supported, particularly English.

(c) Our Relatives Are Bilingual As Well

As we have shown in previous sections, bilingual parents usually discontinued or did not even start using one of their native languages, which meant that their children were not raised trilingually. This section focuses on the impact of the extended family on the language use of this group of trilingual families. We will pay particular attention to grandparents and their language preferences.

Bisera and Drazen

Drazen, a 30-year-old father, spoke Croatian and German as his native languages, while his 27-year-old wife, Bisera, spoke Bulgarian and German. She had grown up in Bulgaria, but had lived and studied in Germany for the previous seven years. Drazen, who worked as a scientist, was born in Germany but had lived the first four years of his life in Croatia before coming back to Germany to stay permanently. The parents spoke German as a lingua franca because they did not understand each other's respective native languages. The couple had one six-month-old daughter, Silke, whom they were hoping to bring up speaking Bulgarian, German and Croatian. However, learning Croatian was not going too well, as Drazen felt that he did not have the necessary time to use this language with his daughter regularly and neither did he feel confident with his identity. Drazen said: 'I feel that when I am in Croatia the environment doesn't accept me as a real Croatian and the same here in Germany where I am not accepted as a real German. I am between two worlds.'

Drazen was also worried that Silke might learn Bulgarian first, which would have disadvantaged German and most of all Croatian. He even became angry when Bisera tried to portray a more positive picture, saying that their daughter would pick up German as the parents spoke it all the time between them. Drazen also thought that his daughter might start speaking Bulgarian with him, which he described as a 'devastating scenario'. In addition, Drazen mentioned the pressure from the Croatian community, who expected him to use Croatian with his daughter. Drazen said:

> When we fly to Croatia I want my daughter to be able to communicate with my relatives. She must be able to communicate and that is – I don't want to say – it's a disgrace but people see it differently there than in Germany. I was talking to a relative two weeks ago and he said it would be a disgrace if your daughter can't understand Croatian when she comes here. Very conservative.

Bisera also wanted to preserve Bulgarian for her daughter's relatives:

> For me the main thing is that our daughter can communicate when she is in Bulgaria, that she understands my parents and relatives. It doesn't matter if she can't speak well; mainly she can cope there and it's normal that she learns our language and culture.

Drazen was hoping that his parents would speak Croatian with their grandchild, but they mixed the languages all the time. It was relevant that Drazen himself spoke German with his parents rather than Croatian. The grandparents had been living in Germany for over 30 years and 'they speak German therefore very well'.

Most of the bilingual parents in Group 2 either came from bilingual countries or were children of immigrants. These parents also had parents (the children's grandparents) who were bilingual, which did not support minority language use with their children. This is significantly different from Group 1 families, where the grandparents were usually monolingual and monocultural, as explained in Chapter 3. Also, most of the grandparents lived in the same country where their grandchildren lived, and they usually preferred speaking the community language there. For example, Radhika, a British/Indian mother living in England, said 'I speak English more than Urdu and my mum [grandmother] understands English as well, so I speak to mum [grandmother] in English'. Another example was given by Ilmi, a Finnish mother living in England, who described the language preferences of her Greek/British parents-in-law (her children's paternal grandparents). They preferred speaking English with their grandchildren rather than their native language. Ilmi said:

> When our children were born we thought that three languages is too much and I wanted them to have a strong English. We decided that he [father] was going to speak Greek initially and I was going to speak English to please his [Greek/British]

parents mainly and his parents obviously weren't supposed to speak English to my children because they should speak Greek to my children. But it turns out they speak English to the children mainly. So this is really annoying and it annoys my husband as well because he really did it for his parents, you know, initially, and they [grandparents] don't even speak Greek [to the children].

There were similar examples where the grandparents did not use their minority language with their children or with their grandchildren. Consequently, the parents seemed to lose their motivation to use both native languages. A key factor in some cases may have been that, because the grandparents were able to communicate with their grandchildren in one language, usually the community language, they preferred the ease of using that language over the longer-term advantages of practising a less preferred language with them. Although most participants mentioned their relatives in some way, only a few actually stated that their relatives were supportive of the parents' maintenance of the home language with their children. One of them was a Mongolian/Russian-speaking family. Dalan, the father, said: 'We also have relatives here. They usually visit us and they also speak of course with my daughter in Mongolian. In this way she is learning Mongolian.'

In most families, however, the relatives who lived in the parents' host country did not use their native languages, but instead preferred speaking the community language. Radhika, a second-generation British/Pakistani mother, said: 'My mum's family lives in the UK and most of my husband's family is here. Our children have cousins and they speak to each other in English.' In this case, the presence of the children's cousins did not support the use of the mother's native language because they preferred to speak the community language with each other. This also applied to the grandparents, who could communicate in the community language with their grandchildren without the need for additional languages.

Summary

Family concerns were an important factor in the commitment that many of the parents in Group 1 made to bringing up their children trilingually (see Chapter 3). Family factors did not have the same impact on parents in Group 2. Most families in this group had at least one set of grandparents who were bilingual, so that, in general, the bilingual parents only had to use one of their two native languages to enable their children to communicate with their grandparents. Most of these grandparents also spoke the language of the community where the children lived, which meant that the parents tended not to use one of their native languages with their children.

The parents commented on the attitudes and influence of other relatives, but few said they were supportive of the parents maintaining their home languages. A Russian/English mother said: 'I wanted her [child] to talk to my family and friends in Russian, so I think, yes, I would consider but like everybody not just the parents alone but the whole family and friends and the whole environment'. When discussing their use of languages with their children, many of the parents in Group 2 did not directly refer to their relatives. It seemed that most of the bilingual parents made decisions about their use of their native languages on the basis of convenience, and they found that one language was often sufficient for the children to communicate with their bilingual grandparents and other relatives.

(d) Cultural Identity and Language Maintenance

So far we have discussed how parents Group 2 described their use of languages with their children, taking account of the children going to school, the language competence of the parents and the language preferences of grandparents. In this final section we will explore parents' accounts of their cultural background and how it had influenced their use of languages with their children. Language is a central feature of human culture. How did parents describe their cultural backgrounds and what part did a desire to pass on their native cultural values and traditions to their children play in their language choices?

Olga and Ambrozy

Olga, a 51-year-old mother, had come to England from her native Russia 15 years earlier. Her husband, Ambrozy, who was the same age, had grown up in England with his Polish parents and spoke English and Polish as native languages. Both parents were working in professional jobs. At a mature age they adopted a one-year-old boy, Sam, who was being brought up bilingually in Russian and English. The father did not use Polish with his son as he wanted to concentrate on English. Ambrozy said:

> We thought we would follow one person one language. Now obviously I couldn't speak Polish to Sam because if I spoke Polish to him and Olga spoke Russian there would be no English and he has to have English as his first language as he lives in England. So my job is English and Olga's is Russian.

When Olga was asked about her cultural background, she said '*I am Russian*'. Nonetheless, she added:

> Ah, of course I have lived in England for 15 years. It's obviously part of my culture nowadays. I came over here to England and now I live here and I am exposed to the English culture every day and obviously I regard it as part of my culture because it's the country I chose to live.

Ambrozy, on the other hand, said that 'in terms of nationality I see myself more British'. He also believed that 'it's impossible to do a language without the culture and without the history'. Furthermore, he felt uncomfortable with the fact that he himself had grown up bilingually: 'I think I was a bit confused having too many languages. I have always felt it was a bit confusing when I was a child.' Although he did not use Polish with his child, he signalled an interest in taking his son to Poland so that he could learn some of the Polish cultural traditions. However, priority was given to the English language. Ambrozy said:

> We should take our son to Poland at some point, ah, and obviously he will speak some Polish but not at the expense of English. If it is at the expense of English then he will find linguistically he doesn't quite know where he is and culturally he doesn't quite know where he is. I think he has got to have a strong identity linguistically and culturally.

The mother too wanted Sam to be British first, as somebody 'who was born and brought up in England'. However, she also wanted to pass on Russian cultural values to him:

> Since Sam is my son I would like him to be exposed to Russian culture and Russian language, as well as practically because foreign languages are extremely useful. It expands your horizons. Mainly it's just I am trying to introduce Sam to Russian culture through the language.

We found that most parents Group 2 wanted to pass on their native cultural values and customs to their children. Bilingual parents often referred to more than one native cultural tradition when they described their background and these parents wanted to pass on their multiple native cultural traditions to their children, even if most of them dropped one of the associated native languages. Palloma, a Spanish/French mother, said: 'So I want to pass to my son the French and Spanish cultural traditions. But, ah, at home we don't speak French.'

Another parent, Hailey, who came from an Italian/US-American family and was now living in Germany, made similar statements about her background. She spoke only English with her children, while she described Italian, her second native language, as 'not useful'. At the same time, she said: 'I always considered myself as Italian. I perceive myself as Italian.' Hailey said:

> The children should recognise that papa [dad] is German and they are German and mum is Italian American. I don't consider myself 100% American because I really grew up with these two cultures as very important in our family. I am not saying my children have to wear their German, American Italian culture on their sleeves but they are aware – I don't think we make a conscious effort and yet they are very much aware that they do come from these three different backgrounds.

Here, Hailey described her two native cultural traditions as 'very important' in her family, yet she used only English with her children. We also found this trend with other bilingual parents who were committed to passing on two or three native cultural traditions to their children, but not necessarily all the associated native languages. This point was emphasised even more strongly for languages that were regarded as less prestigious or useful. One example was Obasi, who lived in Germany and spoke French and Mòoré (a language with over 5 million speakers in Burkina Faso). Obasi said: 'I speak Mòoré and French as my mother tongues'. He also spoke German, English and Jula (another official language of Burkina Faso) as additional languages. Although he did not identify with the French cultural tradition, he used only French with his child, rather than his African languages. When Obasi was asked if he felt French in some way he said:

> No. I feel as an African from Burkina Faso. It was natural. And I feel good when I speak French. The problem is that the official language is French or English. It is better for the future when you speak French or English and when the child speaks French she can integrate more easily in Africa.

His wife, Angelika, who was originally from Germany, added: 'It is also easier for me to learn French through my daughter rather than an African language'.

This, then, was another reason why some bilingual parents did not use their available native languages even though they felt connected to the native cultural traditions of their own childhood. Instead, they spoke a major European language with their children for practical reasons, because of their limited competence in their native language or their perception of its relatively low international status. English in particular enjoys such high prestige that some parents in our study gave up their own native languages in order to bring up their children with a language that they saw as being useful everywhere.

It became clear that bilingual parents were especially likely to identify themselves as bilingual with two languages and two cultures if they had been exposed to both cultures and languages throughout their childhood. Some of these parents, however, had ambivalent feelings about their cultural background. For example, Edwardo, a Spanish/British father, said: 'I'm more European than anything else. But what do I feel deep down? I feel more Spanish than English.' It emerged that he needed to be encouraged by his wife to use Spanish, as he preferred speaking English with his children. Another father, Drazen, who spoke Croatian and German, mainly used German with his daughter, Silke, despite commenting that 'I would never regard myself as German'.

Summary

Thus the cultural description of families in Group 2 proved difficult, because one or both parents in each family generally referred to two native cultural traditions. 'I wouldn't see myself as German or Croatian, but rather as Croatian/German, a mix … I am between two worlds'. Although most bilingual parents were committed to passing on parts of their native cultural traditions and values to their children, they did not necessarily include all the associated languages. In fact, most bilingual parents in the study did not relate their use of languages with their children to the different cultural traditions that they felt an association with. Cultural affiliation and the use of language appeared to be less strongly linked in this group of parents than it was Group 1, described in Chapter 3.

Conclusion

We have described four main factors that appeared to influence the use of languages at home within Group 2 families. One or both parents in each family spoke two native languages, which could include the community language. It emerged that many parents who spoke two native languages used only one of them with their children, partly because it was difficult to use the OPOL method when they had to decide which language to use with their children. It seems that this decision was affected by the parents' relative proficiency in each language rather than by their sense of cultural affiliation.

The parents also reported that there was often a shift away from trilingual practices when the children began to attend school or nursery. In particular, bilingual parents tended to drop one of their native languages when their children started formal education, ceding precedence to the local community language, which they could also speak. In other cases, the parents used only the local community language because they did not think that their minority languages would be useful for their children. Some parents chose to send their children to multilingual or supplementary schools, but they were rare and/or expensive and usually only supported the major European languages, most commonly English. In general, the maintenance of minority languages was not supported by the educational systems in England or Germany, where the overwhelming emphasis was on the local community language. So, most of the children were immersed in the community language in the classroom, playground and neighbourhood, and this situation made it harder for their parents to use their additional native languages with them effectively at home.

We also examined the language preferences of other relatives, especially grandparents. We found that most families Group 2 had at least one set of grandparents who were bilingual. Most of these grandparents also spoke the language of the community where the children lived. This was one of the factors that led bilingual parents to discontinue one of their additional native languages: because the grandparents did not need the children to speak their original native languages, they did not give the parents strong support in their efforts to use or maintain both of their languages at home. This was also true for other relatives, who often spoke the community language and therefore did not support the families' trilingualism.

Finally, most bilingual parents Group 2 did not explicitly link their different cultural traditions with their use of languages with their children. Although they did want to pass on parts of their native cultural traditions and values to their children, such as religious beliefs and ceremonies, food or parenting methods, these values did not usually include all the associated languages. Thus, for most of the bilingual parents, their cultural background outside the country where they were now living did not influence their choice of languages to use with their children. Those decisions were more strongly influenced by practical considerations, such as their proficiency in their additional native languages and their perception of the status and usefulness of those languages. In this context, the parents' bilingual proficiency, and in particular their proficiency in the local community language, acted against the realisation of their children's potential trilingual proficiency.

Further Support for Trilingual Families (Group 2)

Studies, including ours, suggest that committing to one minority language from the beginning is the best way to maintain trilingualism. This will help the child to develop a structured command of the language. There is a good deal of literature (see reference list at the end of this book) suggesting that OPOL is a helpful strategy that prevents language confusion. But this is not always possible for a mother or father who speaks two native languages, as is the case with Group 2 families. They often asked in emails and forums which language they should use with their children. We found that bilingual parents often had a language preference in which they felt culturally and emotionally at home. Perhaps it would be advisable to use that language as a parent and employ, for example, a nanny or multilingual school or nursery to maintain the second minority language (see Chapter 6 for more information on multilingual schooling). It may be valuable when Group 2 families have a minority community in the area offering language clubs or supplementary and complementary language classes. However, this requires effort from the parents and children and is not always desired by trilingual teenagers.

Xiao-lei Wang, a linguist and mother of two trilingual children, has written a number of books for multilingual families, such as *Growing Up With Three Languages: Birth to Eleven* (2008) and *Learning to Read and Write in the Multilingual Family* (2011). She suggests that it can be helpful for parents to use a minority language to cover some of the topics at home which their children have learned in school. For example, if they learned something about photosynthesis, the parents would then discuss the same subject in their minority language after school. Both parents and children may find this strategy tiring and impractical, as children want to play when they come home. But when the children are excited about a topic or go on a school trip or learn about something outside their parents' experience, there may be the basis for a genuine, two-way conversation in one of the minority languages that interests everyone.

Language status seems to be another reason why certain parents struggle with trilingualism. As mentioned earlier, Obasi from Bukina Faso, who lived in Germany, spoke two native languages, French as well as Mòoré, an African language. He would have liked to speak Mòoré with his son but refrained from doing so because he felt this language was not useful or appreciated outside Bukina Faso. His German wife also asked him to use French, because she could speak it. Consequently, Obasi just used French, despite the fact that he did not identify with French culture. Indeed, he felt some resentment towards the language as a reminder of colonial oppression. Still, he normally used French with his children, even though it was not his strongest language. That may mean that he did not give them the best language model of which he was capable, but in Europe, where they were living, he gave more priority to social and economic factors: using French with his children opened doors for them to education, employment and media. Perhaps, if there were more awareness of the benefits of trilingualism in traditionally monolingual societies, parents and educators would see nurturing minority languages as more of a benefit to children's cognitive and social development. Further reading on this and other subjects can be found in Chapter 7 and at the end of the book.

5   One or Both Parents Are Trilingual (Group 3)

Introduction

Our aim in Chapter 5 is to describe the language practices of families in Group 3. This group included a range of different language combinations, usually consisting of at least one parent who spoke three native languages. The two parents always had at least three native languages between them, so that they had the option to bring up their children trilingually.

Figure 5.1 gives a simple overview of Group 3 families (a full review of all the main groups can be found in Chapter 1). In describing this group of trilingual families, we paid attention to the language use of the families and their relatives, as well as to the families' cultural identity. We found that families in this group in England and Germany followed different language patterns with their children. Families in England

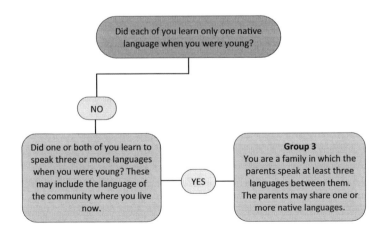

Figure 5.1 Language background tool – Group 3

were much more likely to use only the community language with their children than families in Germany. For that reason, we will examine the differences that were found between parents living in England and those living in Germany in how they explained their language practices. In doing so, we will take into account the impact on their decisions of the status of English as a global language. The following questions are explored in this chapter:

- Why are the language practices of trilingual families in Group 3 in England and Germany different?
- What influence do community attitudes and schooling arrangements have on the families' efforts to maintain their home languages?
- What role do relatives play in the language use of trilingual families in this group?
- How does the cultural background of the families affect their language use?

(a) Trilingual Families and the Use of English

One of the objectives outlined above is to explain trilingualism in England and Germany. Both European countries are officially monolingual, and it was assumed that this would have an influence on trilingual practices within families living there. In addition, English has developed into a global language, and this affected the language maintenance of trilingual families in this study. While families in Groups 1 and 2 showed similar language patterns in both countries (see Chapters 3 and 4), families Group 3 were different. We found that Group 3 families in England were more likely to bring up their children monolingually than parents in Germany. These different language practices were influenced by a number of factors, such as variations in the parents' language background. This group combined families where the parents had different backgrounds with families where one parent was trilingual; the latter represented the largest part of the group in England, where the trilingual parent spoke two languages in addition to English, while their partners spoke only English, as a native language. Maija, an English/Swedish/Finnish-speaking mother, married to John, said: 'I actually came more to the fact that it is so much more natural to speak English with the children'. Therefore, the shared language for most of these families was English, and this was the language of the society in which they were living. This, in the parents' opinion, made it impractical to use other available family languages at home, as the following family example shows.

Rafa and Deon

Rafa was a 43-year-old second-generation British/Pakistani national who came to England in her early teens. Her 46-year-old husband came from the English-speaking part of the West Indies. Both parents were employed as manual workers. They had four boys, aged 26, 25, 22 and 13 years, who were all brought up monolingually, even though the mother was a trilingual speaker of English, Urdu and Punjabi. Rafa said:

> I am able to communicate very well with people from my home background when we come together. We do speak very well fluent in Punjabi and Urdu and English as well. In my own home we really just speak in English most of the time. None of my children or husband speaks other languages.

According to Rafa, it seemed normal for the family to speak English, 'because we both [parents] speak English and plus we live in an English country, it just comes naturally'. The parents did not discuss the subject of language choice before the children were born. The mother felt regretful that the children could not speak her native languages, except for a few Urdu words. However, she did not use her native languages because her husband spoke only English. 'This is, you know, what my husband decided. If the children learnt to speak Punjabi or Urdu then if we communicate my husband will be left out.'

In addition, the maternal grandmother could speak Punjabi and Urdu plus English, as she came from Pakistan to England in the 1950s as an immigrant. The paternal grandmother also lived in England and she spoke only English. Both the maternal and paternal grandfathers had died. According to the interviewees, neither the grandparents nor other members of the extended family objected to the parents' 'one language' approach. Rafa also mentioned that her children's cousins could speak only English: 'All the kids, none of my sister's side, can't speak it [Urdu nor Punjabi], so they all communicate in English you see, so it's only the older people'.

The parents expressed their joy that their children were speaking English so well. When they were asked to comment on their children's English, Rafa answered: 'The children are quite good, set two [second of the highest school grade]'. The parents regarded their own English as 'very good'.

Rafa and Deon represent a typical Group 3 family in England, where both parents spoke English at a native level of proficiency and, in addition, one parent spoke two further native languages. This makes English the dominant language. Looking more closely at the language background of other families in this group, we found that most fathers in the English sample spoke only English. They would have been excluded from conversations if the trilingual mothers had used one of their additional native languages with their children.

In Germany, on the other hand, the linguistic milieu in Group 3 families was different, as there were no families in which both parents spoke the community language, German, as their native language. This made German less accessible in their families, even though it was the language of the community. Instead, the parents employed one of their shared native languages as a lingua franca or the parents used English as a neutral shared non-native language. Among the parents we interviewed, most used at least one native language with their children and encouraged the development of English by sending them to international schools, as the following example shows.

Caroline and Dirk

Caroline, the 40-year-old mother, grew up in Tunisia as the daughter of Italian immigrants who spoke French, Italian and Arabic. Caroline too acquired these three languages, but at the age of eight she stopped using Arabic when the family moved to Haiti. For the last 12 years the mother had been living in Germany, where she had married Dirk, her 43-year-old German husband. They had two boys, aged five and seven years, and a six-year-old daughter. The two younger children were adopted. The children were brought up speaking French, English and German. Dirk spoke German and English with the children, and Caroline spoke French and English with them.

The parents opted for an international school, where the children learnt French, English and German. The parents communicated in English with each other rather than German, the father's native language and the language of the community. 'I speak English to Dirk and he speaks English with me. We very, very seldom speak German together, and when so, only one sentence.' Additionally, the parents opted to use English with their children as a foreign language, besides French and German. Therefore, the mother neglected two of her native languages, Italian and Arabic, and concentrated on French and English. 'I speak French and English to the children. Dirk speaks German and English to the children. In the end, it came naturally.'

Both parents had lived and studied in England, which made English an important language for this family. 'We both love England and most of our friends live there. They are polite and service oriented. We love that.'

The global popularity of the English language and its usefulness for the future as well as the high socio-economic status of most of the parents made English an important language for Group 3 families in Germany. Eckert, a German father, explained why he used English with his children:

I am teaching a lot in English and English is a language which you simply need to know. And I don't want my daughter to speak perfect English but that she gets used to the language early on, so she gets used to the sound. And it's a good training as I don't mind, because I need to teach 50% in English.

Many researchers have pointed to the increasing role of English in multilingual and cross-cultural contexts. It is not only the internet and other media that has contributed to the spread of English, but also the education curriculum in non-English-speaking countries. English is usually the first foreign language in most schools and sometimes it is introduced as early as the preschool stage. Even in international multilingual schools, English is often the medium of instruction. Researchers in multilingualism have become concerned about the dominance of English, as it tends to replace other languages in many contexts and may represent a threat to minority languages.

Summary

Most Group 3 families in Germany added English as a non-native language, because the parents worked or lived in an environment where English was an essential language. Anton, a Serbian father, explained: 'English is very important for our job, so English was always there'. (The next section includes more about Anton's family.) Helmut, a German father, added: 'We are living in an international environment in Germany where English is quite important'. In order to support the children's acquisition of the English language, most families in this group in Germany sought support from international schools to ensure that their children learnt English in an academic environment.

(b) Reported Attitudes Towards Trilingualism in the Community and School

In this section we report what parents in this group had to say about the attitudes of other people in the wider community, including schools. Negative or positive attitudes towards trilingualism in society can have an impact on language use and language learning. For example, when the community attributes negative values to multilingual families' home languages, the community language may replace one or all of the families' native languages. People may be intimidated if their native languages are regarded by the mainstream community or school as 'low status'. We found that most Group 3 families in Germany did report other people having negative attitudes towards trilingualism in children. Bojana, a Macedonian mother, said: 'Most of the people I know they sometimes say "Oh, maybe I don't want to force my child, it's too difficult with two or three languages"'. Other parents also felt that people in the community regarded 'trilingualism as too much'.

These parents, along with all the other families in Germany in Group 3, still raised their children speaking three languages, but that did not necessarily include all available native languages, as the following example shows.

Bojana and Anton

These parents, who were both 39 years old, had been married for 15 years. Anton, the father, worked at the airport, while Bojana was a teacher. After the war had started in the former Yugoslavia, the family migrated to Germany, where they intended to stay. The parents each spoke three native languages, as shown in the following quotation from Bojana:

> When it was ex-Yugoslavia the official language was Serbo-Croatian and I spoke that language. Now it's a separate language, Serbian and Croatian, and I speak both languages and Macedonian because I am Macedonian. So my husband also speaks Croatian, Serbian and Macedonian.

The parents employed Macedonian as a lingua franca between them, although they used increasingly English or German, which they spoke as additional languages. 'English is very important for our job, so English was always there.' Both parents were used to communicating in English as a requirement of their occupation. They had two sons, aged 9 and 14 years, who acquired Macedonian at home, and German and English in a bilingual school, as well as studying Spanish as a subject.

> The children are in English class, which means all the subjects are in English and every day they have German. I mean, when you hear them talking German with a German accent and then you hear them talking English with English accent.

The parents were pleased with their children's progress in school and that they were in a position to acquire several languages:

> Well, I find it really good speaking a few languages ... you can communicate with people. That's why I am happy with my children to speak a few languages and I don't force my children.

The parents in this example had decided to enrol their children in a bilingual English/German school even though English was not a native language for the parents. This meant that they dropped two home languages, Croatian and Serbian. There were other trilingual families who found it difficult to use all home languages, such as Caroline, who was described earlier. She spoke three native languages (Italy, Arabic, French), which were different from the community language. She dropped Italian and Arabic, two of her three native languages. Instead, she used French plus English and German as non-native languages, and these were reinforced for her children through attending a multilingual school. The mother found it impractical to use the OPOL method, as it is intended to support one native language only besides the community language. 'We do not practise OPOL because the theory may sound good but the practice is not always possible.'

In a mainly monolingual society other adults may be puzzled by such a strategy involving three or more languages. The mother felt misunderstood by monolinguals and teachers who, in the mother's opinion, were not in a position to judge a trilingual parent:

> There are what I consider 'Negative monolinguals' who tend to be critical of us: 'No OPOL!! That is bad for the child, it confuses them'. Such comments are made by teachers.

Despite the mostly negative comments, it was found that none of the Group 3 parents in Germany appeared to be intimidated, and none of them said that they modified their language practices with their children because of the perceived attitudes of other people.

The situation with Group 3 families in England was different, since most families raised their children monolingually. Therefore, most of these parents were not in a position to comment on other people's attitudes towards trilingualism in their families. Instead, they reported more general attitudes, as illustrated by a quotation from Maija, a Finnish/Swedish/English-speaking mother:

> A teacher approached me and said: 'There is a language problem. Could that be because you speak Finnish with your son?' And I said: 'Actually, I don't speak Finnish at home'. I was quite cross, because, you know, it's not for a teacher to turn around and say: 'This child may have language problems, therefore you shouldn't be speaking any other language to them', especially if that could be the mother's mother tongue.

Another example is given by Olga, a Russian/Finnish/English mother who only used English with her children:

> If you are in England and you speak a minority language, then it's much more difficult to maintain. I heard that if you are bilingual it takes the children a little longer to sort of getting into the whole situation. But it's a quite superficial thing because the children do catch up quickly.... It slows them down in the beginning, then they pick it all up. So at the beginning it might slow them down in school.

The only Group 3 family in England who raised their children bilingually instead of monolingually reported the attitudes of their neighbours and friends towards their bilingual language practices as both negative and positive. Mirja, an English/Finnish/Swedish/Norwegian-speaking mother, commented:

> Ah, I do get some funny looks I noticed. Everyone, especially my neighbourhood and friends, they all know that I am from Finland and they know that I talk Finnish

to my kids. And some of them actually think 'It's great'; others are sort of like, ah, a bit more negative towards it, why bother, you know. Because I think they don't understand. However, in public and with strangers and then when they hear me talking Finnish, ah, I get funny looks sometimes.

Summary

Thus it becomes clear that the differences in the families' language practices between England and Germany could be attributed, in part, to various factors in the parents' language background. The importance of English as an international language was a significant additional influence. Although the reported attitudes of other people towards multilingualism in both countries were mostly negative, they seem not to have influenced the language choices of parents in this group to a great extent. In the next section we examine the impact of the language knowledge of relatives, in particular of grandparents, on the families' language practices with their children.

(c) The Influence of the Extended Family

As pointed out in the previous section, most Group 3 parents in Germany used English and German with their children. However, they often also employed one of their additional native languages, generally in order to enable their children to speak with the extended family. In fact, half of the grandparents in Germany could not speak the community language, German. Most Group 3 families in Germany reported a link between their language use and their concerns for other relatives, especially grandparents. Aras, a Lithuanian/Russian-speaking father, commented: 'It came from our parents' side that we should use Lithuanian'. Antonelle, an Italian mother, said: 'It would be a catastrophe if my daughter couldn't speak Italian'.

The circumstances in England were rather different, as most of the grandparents and other members of the extended family spoke English very well. This meant that Group 3 parents in England may have used only the community language with their children, partly because the relatives could communicate with the parents and their children in English, without the need for additional languages. Afar, an English/Urdu/Punjabi-speaking father, commented:

> I think my parents, ah, it doesn't really seem to bother them so much that our son Peter doesn't speak Urdu really, because the grandparents have understood what Peter is like as a person. He is actually not willing to communicate with the grandparents if they speak Urdu with him. So, the grandparents would rather have a relationship with him than for Peter not to communicate.

However, one or both sets of grandparents and other relatives in some group 3 families in England spoke only some or no English, which caused communication problems, as the following example shows.

Anais and Irfaan

Irfaan, the 48-year-old father, and Anais, his 35-year-old wife, had been living together for 13 years. They both had Mauritian and British nationality, and both spoke Mauritian Creole and Chinese as their native languages, as well as French and English as additional languages. Irfaan, who worked as a teacher, had been living in England since 1976, and intended to stay. They had two sons, aged eight and five years, who were being brought up speaking mainly English, except for a few words of Mauritian Creole, Chinese and French:

> We speak mostly English, but we do throw in the odd French words or Chinese words and Mauritian words. For example: *boom*, which means apple, *buar*, which is pear. So the children know – once you start to repeat the same words they learn it.

The parents spoke several languages, although it was difficult to define which they spoke as native languages. Mauritian Creole was clearly the strongest language of the parents, as they had been speaking it since their childhood, and they employed it as a lingua franca between them. It was not clear from the interview how well they could speak Chinese. The father only vaguely mentioned that he spoke Chinese because he had a Chinese background; he also mentioned his passion for French literature and that his English was not so fluent. This complex picture of language competence was reflected in the parents' language use with their children.

Using only some words at home seemed to be enough for the father to call his children multilingual. In other words, his understanding of language competence was not measured on fluency but instead on the knowledge of single words. The father thought that 'the child becomes confused, if you have several languages'. When they were in Mauritius, the children had problems with the language, so that they needed people around who understood English as well:

> Ah, they [their sons] would make themselves understood. They say: 'I want this' and then aunty would translate [laughing]. I mean, my mum knows very little English, so she has trouble when she is speaking to my little boys.

There were other families where the grandparents could not speak the community language of their grandchildren. For example, Aira, a Finnish mother, said:

> My dad really doesn't really accept it, because he thinks that the children should be able to speak Finnish and he has complained to me. But his living conditions are very different to ours.

In another example, Uan, a Chinese/Malaysian father, referred to his extended family in Malaysia and China and his wife's family in Finland, including the grandparents, who disapproved of their 'one language' approach:

> When we first visited Finland and obviously both of my daughters did not know Finnish. So when our daughters were in Finland obviously they had difficulties. So it was difficult to play with their cousins or talk to their uncles or aunties.... I think the relatives mind. They actually say: 'Oh shouldn't the children know another language, so when they come that they can speak to the relatives better, easier and understand them better.' It's true, I think there is some sort of a wish that the relatives think: 'Oh why can't the children speak better Chinese or Finnish.'

Nonetheless, some parents thought that they 'don't see the extended family very often', that is, not often enough to implement multilingual language use, or they did not consider their relatives' needs as a good reason to use their native languages with their children. Olga, a Russian/Finnish/English-speaking mother, said: 'I don't care because the relatives are not very close'. Some other families wanted their children to 'have an established language first, so they can learn better after that. So the children would not get so confused.'

Summary

In England, most of the grandparents were able to talk to their grandchildren in English, without the need for additional languages. There were only a few families where the grandparents could not speak English and therefore were unable to communicate with their grandchildren. In Germany, on the other hand, most grandparents could not speak German. Therefore, the parents in this group used at least one native language besides English and German with their children in order to enable them to communicate with their grandparents.

(d) Cultural Background and Language Use

As explained above, the parents Group 3 had a range of different individual language backgrounds. In this section, we explore how they described the impact of their cultural backgrounds on their use of languages with their children. We will look at the degree to which parents felt committed to pass on their native cultural customs and traditions to their children. We will also explore whether the parents' cultural background had some influence on their language use with their children.

There is good reason to assume that the cultural context or sociolinguistic environment of multilingual families plays a role in children's acquisition of second and third languages. In earlier chapters, we have shown that the cultural background of Group 1 parents (Chapter 3) had greater influence on their language choices with their children than was the case for parents in Group 2 (Chapter 4). This section looks at the cultural background of parents as a possible factor in the different language practices of Group 3 parents living in England and their German counterparts. The following trilingual family living in Germany illustrates the issue.

Rasa and Aras

Rasa, the 26-year-old mother, had left Lithuania for Germany 10 years earlier, and Aras, the 33-year-old father, followed two years later to study and work in Germany with the intention to stay. To their 16-month-old son, Alex, and with each other, they spoke a mix of Russian and Lithuanian, although occasionally they used German too. According to the father, the parents spoke Russian and Lithuanian very well. In addition, Rasa spoke German on a native level because she had acquired it in Germany when she was still a youth. Alex was just beginning to use a few words, like 'mama' and 'papa'. The father was slightly concerned about Alex's linguistic ability:

I'm a bit worried when Alex goes to kindergarten that his German is behind, because we only speak Russian and Lithuanian at home.... We have decided, because it came from our parents' side, that we should use Lithuanian and we also thought it's fine if it works, but I am not convinced yet if it works.

Aras also complained that, at the moment, they were speaking Russian too much, because the maternal grandmother, who mainly spoke Russian, was staying with the family in Germany. The maternal grandmother's language preference for Russian also played a role in the mother's national identity. When Rasa was asked about her identity she said: 'I am a Russian girl who was born in Lithuania. Because I talk to my mum in Russian.'

The father, on the other hand, identified more with the Lithuanian part of his background: 'I thought and think that I am Lithuanian'. During the Lithuanian national movement in the early 1990s, the father's Russian name was changed to the Lithuanian equivalent. Both parents referred to their Russian and Lithuanian background. Aras added, 'I try to adapt here [Germany] as much as I can'.

Finally, the parents felt that the community expressed negative attitudes towards their family's trilingualism: 'Some said it's too much.... "Three languages. Oh my god, the poor child!"' However, they agreed on the continuing use of both home languages plus German. (There is more information on this family in Chapter 7.)

This family is typical of many Group 3 families in Germany, as they were committed to bringing up their children with three languages and three cultural traditions. Although some parents raised concerns about their children's language development, they were determined to overcome these obstacles. The majority of these parents wanted their children to learn about their own cultural traditions and also the cultural values and customs of Germany.

We heard about quite different language and cultural practices from parents in trilingual families who lived in England. Here, most parents just used English with their children, ignoring at least two possible home languages. The following example illustrates a typical Group 3 family living in England.

Maija and John

Maija, a 35-year-old English/Swedish/Finnish-speaking mother, shared English as a common native language with John, her 36-year-old monolingual English husband. The parents had been living together in England for 19 years. The family never intended to stay in England but they had an autistic child, which they felt made it difficult to move to another country. The mother said:

> My mother is English, my father is [a] Swedish-speaking Finn.... I was brought up speaking in English with my mother. When the whole family were together we spoke Swedish. I went to a Swedish school but obviously all my friends were Finnish, so I spoke Finnish with kids.

The parents had a five–year-old daughter and a seven-year-old son, who were being brought up speaking only English. Maija thought that speaking English with her children was more natural. She commented: 'Fostering closeness and bonding with your children is the most important thing and I do believe that has to be what you consider your mother tongue'. The mother described her daughter's English as 'absolutely excellent'. The family also went to a Finnish school twice a month for one hour, where the daughter could listen to the 'language [and] the intonation'. At the same time, the mother was very pessimistic about her children's chance to learn her native languages:

> I think the problem in this country is we don't hear Finnish or Swedish; we don't really mix with a lot of Finnish or Swedish people or enough that the children would be getting continual feedback. So the times I had tried to speak Finnish would be at bathtime, when I'm singing Finnish and Swedish songs to them, but there are no natural times of the day.

Maija described herself as 'more Finnish than English because obviously the formative years were in Finland.... And also your language is the culture, it actually shows the culture.' The mother also wanted to pass on her native cultural values to her children, because she regarded them as 'part' of herself:

> If my children don't have the culture then they don't understand [that] part of me. I want to have a summer cottage. I want to keep it there [in Finland].

> And also they [the children] have passports. I have given them the option. When they are 18 they can choose. So I want them to have a choice, and to enable them to have a choice obviously I have to give them [the children] a background.

There were many such families in our study where the trilingual parent wanted to pass on cultural values to the children, but without prioritising the native languages. As a consequence, the children learnt only English. Balanced trilingualism is difficult to achieve. The use of home languages seems particularly difficult when the parents have no language support from the community or other family members. In addition, when the couple share the community language as a native language, it may be even harder to use additional languages in the family.

We found that most Group 3 mothers and fathers in England regarded it as important to pass on their native cultural values and traditions to their children. In general, these values concerned foods, religious ceremonies, clothing or respecting older people. However, it seems that language was not included as a cultural marker because most parents in this group of families in England raised their children monolingually, by dropping the associated native languages. For example, one family spoke more than three native languages between them: Finnish (mother), and Punjabi, Urdu and Hindi (father), as well as the community language, English. Amir, the father, regarded himself as 'Asian, Asian Christian', while Aira, the mother, rejected the English culture quite strongly: 'I have never considered myself English and I never will be'. Despite the rejection of 'English' cultural values, both parents in this family spoke only English with each other and with their children.

There were other such families in our study, for example Anais and Irfaan, who described their cultural background as 'Chinese' and who referred to four languages: 'We are fluent in English, French, mother tongue is Pidgin French [Mauritian Creole] and as having a Chinese background we also speak Chinese'. Uang, another Chinese father, described his cultural background as 'Chinese' and 'Buddhist', although he grew up in Malaysia: 'You have to learn Malaysian culture. It's a very cosmopolitan culture. It's a mix, because in Malaysia you have over 55% Malay and 30% Chinese about.' Although these two families spoke many languages and dialects, they used only English with their children, as did most of the other Group 3 parents in England. Many of these parents reported mixed identities, as the following quotations show:

- Olga, a Russian/Finnish/British mother: 'I have a very confused identity. I mean I just feel that I am a citizen of the world.'
- Maija, a Finnish/British mother: 'I see myself as European. Somebody specifies it then I would say I am half and half, English and Finnish.'
- Uang, a Chinese/British/Malaysian father: 'I am a Chinese, also I am still Malaysian'

- Mirja, a Finnish/American mother: 'My cultural background is more a mixture.'
- Afar, a Pakistani/British father: 'I think I am a mixture of Asian and British'

However, although the parents frequently referred to themselves as having more than one cultural tradition, they only used one language, English, with their children.

Turning to the Group 3 parents in Germany, their language practices were very different from the English sample, in that all the families raised their children trilingually. However, most of the parents employed English as a non-native language, partly because it was an important language for them. In terms of their cultural background, most mothers and fathers wanted to pass on aspects of their native cultural values and traditions to their children. Even though they were living in Germany, some of the families also identified with English cultural values through the language when they described their cultural background. Pavlov, a Czech/Dutch father said: 'I would say that we probably identify more with English, so probably English first, Dutch second, German third'. Another example is given by Caroline, a French/Italian/Tunisian mother, who had lived 10 years in England before coming to Germany 11 years earlier.

> French are more spontaneous, but then again my German husband is rather spontaneous. Germans like to follow rules, but then again I learnt it has advantages. English, oh! We both love England and most of our friends live there.... We want our children to learn the best of all three cultural traditions and more.

Summary

Most of the families in this group were committed to passing on their home cultural values to their children, but they did not necessarily think that it meant they should pass on the associated home languages. The cultural background of the Group 3 families in England and Germany did not have as much influence on their use of languages with their children as we had found with Groups 1 and 2. Instead, there were other factors that seemed more significant in their decisions about this, notably the importance of English as a global language and the concerns of grandparents.

Conclusion

This chapter has explored four main factors affecting the language practices of families in Group 3, the smallest group in this study – language competence, education, relatives and culture. There were major differences in language practices between families in this group living in England and those living in Germany. A key factor that affected the parents' language choices was language background. For example, in most families in England both parents spoke the community language, English, as one of their native languages, or alternatively the parents had lived in an English-speaking country for over 20 years and therefore they spoke English at a high level. That may explain to some degree why most parents in England used only the community language with their children, as English was the shared language for most of the couples.

In contrast, there was no family in the German sample where both parents spoke the community language, German, as their native language. Consequently, they used one of their shared native languages or English with their children. Moreover, most Group 3 families in Germany enrolled their children in international schools that included English, even though this language was not spoken as a native language by the parents. The popularity of the English language and its usefulness for the future were the main reasons for choosing English as a non-native language. As a result, the parents neglected at least one home language. For example, Pavlov regarded Czech, his additional native language, as not valuable for their children: 'I consciously made the choice to use English, which would be the most useful for the children in the future'.

Other parents in Group 3 even neglected two home languages, such as Caroline, a trilingual mother who dropped Italian and Arabic. Instead, she was speaking in French and English with her children, ignoring the OPOL method because she found it impractical: 'We do not practise OPOL because the theory may sound good but the practice is not always possible'. In most cases the parents had a high socio-economic status, which required speaking English at work, which added to that language's importance in the family, as pointed out by Eckert, a German father: 'English is a language which you simply need to know'.

Additionally, most parents in Germany used at least one native language besides English and German with their children in order to enable them to communicate with their grandparents, who generally could not speak German. In England, on the other hand, most of the grandparents in this sample of families spoke English, so that they were able to talk to their grandchildren without the need for additional languages. Moreover, we found that, although most of the families in Germany reported that other people in the community had negative attitudes towards trilingualism, all of them raised their children trilingually. Indeed, it appeared that none of the parents allowed their trilingual family practices to be affected by the perceived negative attitudes of other people. In contrast, trilingual Group 3 families in England could not comment on the community's attitudes towards trilingualism in their families, because most of them raised their children monolingually. Instead, they reported more general attitudes towards foreign cultures and languages in England, which most of these parents perceived as negative. But, as in Germany, there was no evidence in what the parents themselves said that these negative attitudes influenced their language choices.

Lastly, the parents' testimonies suggested that their cultural background only partly influenced their use of languages with their children. Even though most Group 3 parents in both England and Germany wanted to pass on their native cultural values and traditions to their children, they did not necessarily think that it needed to include all the associated native languages. Many parents in this group regarded certain cultural markers as more important than language, such as 'fostering closeness and bonding with your children', certain foods or religious beliefs and ceremonies. So the differences in language practices between the parents in England and Germany were only partly influenced by their wish to pass on their native cultural traditions and values. Other factors played a more important role, as outlined in this chapter.

Recommendations for Trilingual Families (Group 3)

Trilingual families in which at least one parent speaks three languages have great difficulty in bringing up their children to speak three languages when they live in mainly monolingual countries. As this chapter shows, the parents really struggle with tri-lingualism because of language competence challenges and practical issues. No specific strategies have a strong evidence base in mainly monolingual societies. In Chapter 6 we show that many people learn to use three languages competently in countries where trilingualism is the norm. Here, typically, each language is used in a different context. But the context for a trilingual family in Group 3 in a mainly monolingual country is quite different, with the influence of the community language being much stronger. However, some of the suggestions given for Group 1 and Group 2 families may partly work for Group 3 families in this situation. For example, enrolling children in supple-mentary or multilingual schools and nurseries (see Chapter 6 for more information on multilingual schooling) can support one or in some rare instances two minority languages. But, because the parents usually share one native language, they often end up raising their children monolingually or, at most, bilingually. For example, Olga, who was raised speaking Russian and Finnish and also acquired English to a native level in an international school in Finland, explained her struggle:

> Well I speak English to the children. I've got a couple of nursery rhymes in Russian that I sing to them but I know I should speak…. But if you are in England and you speak a minority language then it's much more difficult to maintain it, es-pecially when your spouse is English and you speak English at home. I know some people who manage to speak two languages to their children – so the father speaks English and the mother speaks Finnish…. But that's just not me. I can't see how it should work in our family [sad voice] and for me communication in general is more important.

Some trilingual parents may choose not to use the community language with their children and instead concentrate on a home language. Here the children have the opportunity to become at least bilingual. For example, Maik, a German/French/English-speaking father, and his English-speaking wife lived in Germany. Maik decided to use English with his wife and daughter when they were together. The parents hoped that their young child would learn German in school later on, as the main language of instruction. Maik would then switch to German for homework, while his wife would help with the English assignments. The father also tried to use French, but he seemed to struggle with his efforts. At the end of the research interview Maik resumed: 'I hope we can manage it in a way that our daughter speaks at least German and English'. In this context the child will learn two languages in a balanced way. It is important that parents make informed choices that are practical and workable. It is not desirable that a language is imposed forcefully only for the sake of trilingualism. Often cultural habits and bonding are more important than the language.

Most parents in our study based their choice of language on a sort of instinctive natural reflex, preferring their strongest language. However, this could change, and often did, as trilingual families seem to be more likely to move between countries than their monolingual counterparts. In these circumstances trilingualism is dynamic and constantly adapting to evolving circumstances. We live in an increasingly globalised world, where language contact is becoming the norm. But it seems that minority and low-status languages are not benefiting from this development. Trilingual parents have turned to the internet and internet forums to find support for their language situation. In the following chapters we will give an overview of the extensive resources that deal with issues raised in this and previous chapters.

6 Trilingual Proficiency in a Multilingual Society

Introduction

Other chapters of this book have concentrated on what it is like for children and parents when they develop trilingual proficiency in a mainly monolingual society. In this chapter we are going to consider the rather different situation of children and families in trilingual communities. When children develop knowledge of three or more languages in a country such as England, France, Russia, Japan or Germany, it is usually the result of family migration: one or both of their parents brought another language from elsewhere when they moved to their current mainly monolingual society. In contrast, when a child is born into a community in which there is widespread multilingualism, they will see personal multilingualism as natural and normal, in fact what is expected of them. Three predominantly trilingual communities are given as examples below. It will be seen that a history of group migration or colonial influence may determine the conditions under which a society becomes trilingual and the circumstances that favour 'natural multilingualism' in an area. The location of a territory next to major language blocks may be another factor, especially if there is a commitment to maintaining a unique political and cultural identity that is distinct from those of the dominant neighbours.

Examples of Trilingual Communities

The use of three languages by the Circassian community in Israel

The Circassians were the oldest indigenous people of the north Caucasus. In the late 19th century they were expelled after a Russian invasion. After a troubled period, a large group of them were settled in two small villages in an area that later became Israel. They have preserved their language and cultural heritage since then, while finding an accommodation with the Israeli state as a loyal group of Muslim citizens. Children learn to speak Circassian (Abkhaz-Adyghe) as their mother tongue and home language. Then, depending on where they live in Israel, they acquire Arabic and Hebrew in succession. Arabic is seen as the language of religion and, for those living in one of the villages, as the best language for communication with those in their immediate environment. Hebrew is learned as a second school language and as the language of the wider society.

The use of three languages in Mauritius

Although Mauritius is close to the East African coast, it differs from nearby African countries in that the majority ethnic group is of Indian descent (68%), almost three times larger than the Creole group of African descent. However, language use by children does not appear to vary between ethnic groups. Individuals in the various communities differ in their language use, but the most common pattern is that children learn to speak Creole, French and English and use all three. The Creole, which is strongly influenced by French, is the dominant language for informal conversations and is spoken in over two-thirds of all homes. The second language for most people is French, which is used by teachers of young children and across the mass media. From kindergarten onwards, it is taught as a subject as well as being used as a medium of education. Although English is the sole official language of Mauritius, it is not extensively used as a community language.

The use of three languages in Luxembourg

Luxembourg is a small country with just over half a million inhabitants, located between Belgium, France and Germany. An unusually high proportion of residents (over 40%) are migrants from other countries. Three languages are recognised in law – Luxembourgish (*Lëtzebuergesch*), French and German. In the period after the Second World War Luxembourgish was generally used as the language of speech, both in everyday conversations and in public contexts such as parliamentary debates, while French and German were used for written communication. Over the last 30 years greater use has been made of written Luxembourgish. That may have been partially motivated by an aspiration to preserve a national identity in an increasingly internationalised territory that hosts major institutions of the European Union and global financial companies. At the same time, French (and also English) are used more often in everyday spoken exchanges for effective communication with the growing numbers of non-native residents, though this does not apply universally.

Multilingualism cannot easily be imposed on a population. A national policy that proclaims three official languages may not be reflected in personal multilingualism among that country's children. In Switzerland, for example, the three main languages, French, German and Italian, are each associated with one part of the country, and few children speak all three. There is a fourth official language, Romansch, which is spoken by less than 1% of the population. However, research by François Grin in the 1990s indicated that almost two-thirds of Swiss native French speakers had only limited or no competence in German. A similar proportion of Swiss native German speakers had that level of competence in French. The knowledge of Italian among both groups was even weaker (see Grin, 1995). It may be a multilingual country but monolingual preferences influence how children are brought up.

Another example of this phenomenon is Singapore, which has four official languages – Malay, Chinese, Tamil and English. Here the separation is not territorial but ethnic. There is a policy of bilingual education in schools, and all students learn through English as the medium of instruction. But they are also taught the language of their ethnic background, referred to as their 'mother tongue'. Officially Malay is designated as the national language, but it has a mainly symbolic role. It is used in the national anthem but it is not taught to non-Malays in school. As in many ex-colonial countries, English has become the dominant working language throughout the country, as it has the advantages that it is recognised as a global language and is neutral between ethnic groups. It is the only language taught in all schools at all levels. Most adult citizens are thus bilingual, in the preferred language of their ethnic group and in English.

In many multilingual societies the languages of the country structure a social hierarchy and only elite groups have access to all of them. It is still common in parts of Africa, for example, for an ex-colonial language to be used for government and administration while a shared national language is used as a lingua franca across groups and local indigenous languages in each area. In 2004 Carol Benson studied trilingualism in Guinea-Bissau, a small country that lies between Senegal and Guinea. There are at least 30 indigenous languages spoken locally. Creole, known as Kiriol, is used in many informal settings and the ex-colonial language, Portuguese, is used in schools and in official communications. However, it is reported that only 14% of the population speak Portuguese and less than half speak Kiriol. Many people are bilingual with proficiency in a local language and in Kiriol, but few are trilingual with Portuguese as well. The majority of the trilingual speakers live in the capital city, Bissau, and appear to be members of the national elite.

It will be clear that trilingual and multilingual societies vary a great deal. So there is also variation in children's experiences of learning languages and parents' experiences of supporting them to do so. In many trilingual societies, most children learn to speak either one or two languages at home and in the community, and later learn a second and/or third at school (as in the example of Mauritius, described above). When children use more than one language, it serves a function in their everyday lives, making communication with others more effective. The advantage that is conferred is sometimes purely personal, such as being able to talk to members of their extended family in the country of origin of one of their parents. Sometimes the motivation is economic or professional, such as learning the language of the national elite in order to have access to higher education or a professional career or a salaried post in the national civil service.

Sometimes the motivation will be politically inspired, as in the sponsorship by the Sri Lankan government of a 'Year of Trilingualism' in 2012, shortly after the end of the long civil war. This was intended to encourage people to speak both national languages – Sinhala and Tamil – and to promote English as a common link language. Within 10 years, it was hoped, Sri Lanka would become a nation of three languages – Sinhala, Tamil and English. It was anticipated that this would reduce the ethnic tensions in the country, which are thought to have been exacerbated by language barriers.

However, national policies of this kind are likely to be effective only if the conditions for using three languages exist for citizens at an individual level. If communities have little social or commercial contact, they may continue to exercise what appear to be largely monolingual preferences, even if many have bilingual or trilingual competence. At an earlier stage, if there is no strong personal reason for children to learn three languages and use them, they will not do so.

Claudine Kirsch of the University of Luxembourg made a close study of how six 'ordinary' eight-year-old native Luxembourgish pupils addressed language learning over a period of one year. Living in a multilingual society, all the children understood the importance of learning languages (see Kirsch, 2006). Readers of Kirsch's report in an English-speaking country, such as the UK or the USA, will note the contrast with the schools in their own societies, where the confidence of being native speakers of the global language notoriously makes pupils 'lazy' about learning a foreign language. The children whom Kirsch observed appreciated that they needed languages other than their native Luxembourgish in order to function in Luxembourg, particularly French, which is used for official purposes in the state. But understanding that did not appear to create a real interest in learning French. Kirsch concluded:

> While children had some immediate needs to use German and English, this was not the case with French. As far as German and English is concerned, all children were eager to watch popular movies, listen to songs, read magazines and share information with friends. In addition, they were keen to communicate with German and English speaking non-nationals. In order to participate in socially valued activities and to successfully communicate with acquaintances, the six children endeavoured to use, and thus to learn, these languages.

In the case of French, in contrast, even though it was one of the dominant languages in their country, they needed to use it less often.

> They felt that they had a choice to use or to avoid the language. For instance, they would only watch French television programmes if there were no alternatives and they would only speak French in the presence of an adult if they were required to do so. Even in the French lessons where the use of French was expected, they

tried to get by in Luxembourgish whenever possible. In situations where French was required in shops or restaurants most children preferred to use their parents as mediators.

Two of the six children had a different approach to the use of French, however:

Monique had to use French in her ballet classes and on the rare occasions the family visited French speaking friends. Anne had been socialised into the use of French early on. Her mother had simply refused to speak for her daughter when she knew that the latter had the necessary vocabulary to get by or if she could provide her with the necessary vocabulary. She explained: 'When Anne was able to say 's'il-vous-plait', she was also able to say 'un coca s'il-vous-plait' [a coke please]. I have not ordered her any drinks since she has been able to say that. I simply expect her to make the effort and speak. Some years ago, she thought that she was forced to speak but now she endeavours to speak. At the age of 10, Monique and Anne were now confident enough to converse while their four friends tended to have brief exchanges in French using formulaic phrases.

Kirsch suggested that key reasons behind their reluctance to speak French included a lack of confidence and the fear of making mistakes. But when they felt a need to use a language, they would create opportunities to learn it, paying particular attention to what people said, memorising unknown words and asking for translations. They might ignore opportunities to use a language and interpret others positively to suit their own needs.

The use of particular languages is very often associated with particular settings: a child may use one language at home or in the school playground and another in the classroom, or may be expected to shift from one language in the classroom in the early years to another language of instruction at a later stage of schooling. However, the picture may be more complex and sometimes quite confusing. For example, in Orissa in eastern India the official language is Oriya. In addition, English is the language of education and administration as well as being used as the shared language in some multilingual situations. But children are exposed to Hindi extensively in the mass media, so that they learn Hindi too from an early age. So children in urban settings grow up learning all three languages simultaneously. But, when Smita Sinha of Berhampur University observed first-grade students in a number of private schools in the capital city, she found that, while they spoke only English in the classroom, their informal conversations in the playground involved extensive language mixing (see Sinha, 2009). What was immediately remarked by a linguistics researcher was that they did not show the consistent patterns of moving between languages at particular points in a sentence or for particular purposes that have been observed in many other countries. They switched codes between Oriya, English and Hindi as though they had them in their minds as a single code. Sinha thought they seemed to be unaware of how much and in what ways they were switching between languages and thought of their mixed languages as a single code. It may be relevant that many urban parents in Orissa in elite groups speak to their children in English along with Oriya and that some parents also mix codes while talking to their children.

In some trilingual settings language mixing of similar complexity seems to arise because parents come from different regions. One example of this is the Aran Valley in the Spanish Pyrenees, where people speak Aranese, the local variant of Gascon, as well as Catalan, the regional language, and Castilian Spanish, the national language. With improved transport opportunities the population is much more mixed than it was when the valley was more isolated. In the course of their research, Jordi Suils and Angel Huguet interviewed young men about their language use. One of them said: 'I talk Castilian to my father and Aranese to my mother depending on who I am looking at while talking'. The researchers commented that it is possible for these trilinguals to start a conversation in one of the three languages and then switch to another one even within a sentence (see Suils & Huguet, 2001). The presence of significant numbers of monolingual Spanish speakers with whom everyone uses Spanish created a slow shift in which that language was building a dominant position. The political revival of Catalan amid growing pressures for Catalonian autonomy and an increasing demand for the protection of Aranese have challenged that dominance, but, as elsewhere, such imbalances between languages are not easy to change.

Across the world, an important factor in children's learning and use of multiple languages is their perception of the status of each of the languages that are available to them. In some countries, such as Guinea-Bissau, trilingualism is associated with high social status. Voluntary trilingualism has a different status in most societies that are mainly monolingual. In European societies, such as England and Germany, many bilingual and trilingual speakers are seen by the majority as having low social status – as immigrants and refugees from poorer parts of the world. Bojan, a teacher and translator who is originally from Serbia but now lives in Germany, said:

> When other people are around and we speak Serbo-Croatian then they react a bit strange, they find it a bit … I wouldn't say naughty but different…. Friends have expressed their dissatisfaction but I am used to it.

Schooling in a Multilingual Context

As we showed in earlier chapters, the linguistic environment of the school may be an important factor in the outcome for individual children. In a study reported in 2010, Viktorija Ceginskas interviewed 12 adults of multilingual and multicultural backgrounds. They were all multilingual in the sense that they had grown up hearing and speaking several languages from birth and were still using a number of languages either in private (with their family and friends) or in their work, although not necessarily on a daily basis. They ranged in age from their early 20s to their early 50s and they had spent their childhood and adolescence in Europe, South and North America and Asia. They were now living in northern Europe and were interviewed at their homes in Sweden, Germany, the Netherlands and Belgium. The seven informants who had exclusively attended local state schools highlighted negative feelings about their multilingualism. One said: 'We're not Swedes, not Estonians, not Lithuanians. We're nothing. We are nothing!' At school they had tended to feel conspicuous, strange and alien, as if they were unique, even when there were other multilingual pupils in the school. They reported that their exchanges with multilingual and multicultural peers were very limited. So they found multilingualism an exotic and difficult experience. Ceginskas suggested that their negative experiences could have been influenced by the fact that their family languages were less commonly used in their dominant environment, and therefore less valued. Moreover, they had attended school in the early phases of the recent process of globalisation, and the situation might be more favourable now. However, the school environment could have made a positive difference even then.

A contrasting subgroup in Ceginskas's sample showed a different attitude, seeing multilinguality as a bonus that had added to their personal experience. One said:

> I grew up in a bubble and that bubble was full of people who were kind of like me, meaning had parents from different nationalities away from the place they lived in, spoke a couple of languages if not more. It was a completely normal experience.

They had not felt strange or different because they had interacted regularly with others who were like themselves from early on, either with multilingual, transnational family friends or in school, most notably in European or international schools. They were accustomed to meeting and mixing with other bicultural/multicultural and bilingual/multilingual people. Within their peer group the complex identity of the multilingual speaker was understood and accepted by others. Such schools could be said to create a multilingual island in societies that are having difficulty in moving away from a largely monolingual heritage. Many urban state schools in northern Europe now aspire to develop that ethos in a way that was probably not possible when the adults who spoke to Ceginkas went to school. This aspiration is exemplified in the association for early multilingualism in day nurseries and schools in Germany (Frühe Mehrsprachigkeit an Kitas und Schulen – FMKS). The association promotes multilingualism in children through immersion programmes and informs parents about multilingual education options. Most of the schools and nurseries that are promoted are publicly funded and emphasise a particular language, such as Polish, Italian, Danish, French or English. Researchers, such as Ofelia García, Tove Skutnabb-Kangas and Maria E. Torres-Guzman, have examined the pedagogical, socio-educational and socio-political aspects of multilingual schools. They have highlighted literacy development in minority languages, multi-identity development and mother tongue support as some of the key benefits of multilingual schools (see García et al., 2006).

The development of 'European schools'

The creation of the European Union (EU) was intended, among other strategic priorities, to facilitate travelling and working across national borders within the group of countries that had come together. In support of this goal, new language policies came into force. The European Union has 24 official and working languages: Bulgarian, Croatian, Czech, Danish, Dutch, English, Estonian, Finnish, French, German, Greek, Hungarian, Irish, Italian, Latvian, Lithuanian, Maltese, Polish, Portuguese, Romanian, Slovak, Slovene, Spanish and Swedish. While the European Commission limits its language use to English, French and German, the European Parliament includes all 24 official languages when needed. At an early stage it was recognised that this policy required the children of migrant workers within Europe to maintain and develop the languages of their country of origin and to acquire a high standard of proficiency in one or more other European languages. To this end, European schools were established to provide education for children with different mother tongues and nationalities.

The main aim of these schools is to promote multilingualism and multiculturalism in the EU. The first European school began in 1953 in Luxembourg, initiated by the European Coal and Steel Community. It was to be a school where children of parents with different nationalities studied in their mother tongue. It quickly became a success academically and other countries followed, such as Belgium, Italy, Germany, Netherlands and the UK. Now there are 14 European schools offering education from nursery level to university entrance. In each school, basic instruction is given in the official languages of the EU, 'to safeguard pupils' mother tongues'. Some of the main objectives are to give pupils confidence in their cultural identity, sound education in the mother tongue and two or more foreign languages, based on a broad range of subjects.

Many people across Europe have learned to be sceptical of worthy but potentially ineffective EU initiatives. How has this one fared when subjected to scholarly investigation? In a doctoral thesis project at Oxford University, Nicola Savvides interviewed teachers and students at three of the schools (in England, Belgium and Spain). The teachers were keen that they should not be seen as 'political tools to turn out "perfect Europeans"'. But they did aim to encourage a European perspective through cross-national comparisons of the topics studied in class. From the perspective of the pupils, however, Savvides concluded that the most influential factor was the many opportunities offered by the schools for pupils of different European backgrounds to interact with one another. They learned a great deal about each other and, in that context, also reflected on 'their own multiple, hybrid identities'. In the setting of the schools, national stereotypes were challenged, and many students developed some of the language skills, social skills and open-minded attitudes that are a prerequisite of a European or global citizen (see Savvides, 2008).

When Mary Hayden and Jeff Thompson of the University of Bath compared the opinions of students at European schools with those of students at other international schools in Europe and in other parts of the world, they found some differences in the prevailing views of each group. The students at the European schools attached a high level of importance to speaking more than one language fluently and to being in a school environment where a number of languages were spoken. While students in all three groups rated the speaking of fluent English as very important, those in European schools gave a higher priority to general language proficiency and to a multilingual environment. Thus they tended to support the policy of their schools that subjects should be studied through more than one language and that students should learn to speak the local language of the country where the school was situated (which was markedly less common in international schools) (see Hayden & Thompson, 1997).

Making Sense of Multilingualism

It will be clear that the expression of multilingual skills is very complex in everyday life, in education, and in commerce and politics. All the factors that influence how bilingual speakers use their two languages come into play, but other factors operate too, because of the multiple possibilities for interactions between three or more languages. Sometimes, as in Guinea-Bissau, trilingual proficiency has been the property of an elite; sometimes, as in the Circassian villages in Israel, it has been universal but restricted to a very small community. Everywhere, the conditions for communal support for trilingualism depend on the political context, such as the goal of social renewal after a civil war in Sri Lanka or the maintenance of ethnic balance in Singapore or the survival of a small nation state amid larger neighbours in Luxembourg. We cannot understand trilingualism simply in terms of a speaker having monolingual-like competence in three languages. It is not even helpful to think of the development of 'balanced trilingualism' in the way that linguists often describe 'balanced bilingualism': a straightforward equality in an individual's use of three or more languages is rare. A speaker's vocabulary or the use of syntax or sensitivity to the nuances of a language will differ between the languages that make up that speaker's multiple repertoires. They may have mastered the language and speech registers of school usage in one language, of the office in another and of the kitchen, the dining room and the bedroom in a third. What matters for individuals is that they have the total linguistic proficiency to communicate with all those with whom they want and need to communicate. The French Canadian linguist Francois Grosjean argued that the language competence of bilingual speakers should not be regarded as just the sum of two monolingual competences but should instead be judged as an overall communicative competence, aspects of which will come to the fore in different social situations. The analogy he uses is of a hurdler (see Grojean, 1985). A sprinter can run faster on the flat and a high-jumper can jump higher, but neither has the unique combination of skills that enables a hurdler to race so fast over obstacles. Bilinguals switch between their languages flexibly for a variety of reasons. They may simply be meeting the needs of those with whom they are talking if they are monolingual, or, if they share the same bilingual competence, they may be seeking to convey emphasis or intimacy or private meanings. Grosjean was writing about bilingualism, but his account applies equally to trilingualism.

Larissa Aronin of the University of Haifa in Israel and Muiris Ó Laoire of Auckland University of Technology in New Zealand have suggested that it will be helpful to understand the patterns of language use among multilingual speakers if we think of the 'dominant language constellations' that affect them. They argue that multilingualism has three main constituents – the languages, the environment and the speaker. Like Grosjean, they aim to focus on the whole set of languages as a unit rather than on one of the languages used by an individual or a group of people. What they term 'multilinguality' involves more than just knowledge of three or more languages: it is intertwined with many aspects of a person's identity or that of a whole group, including their cultural awareness, their attitudes and their social ties and influences. The growth and maintenance of trilingualism can be understood through metaphors from ecology. The changing mix of different languages in an individual's development or a society's history can be thought of as constituting a kind of ecosystem, subject to natural forces that trigger fluctuation, input, absorption and decay. They emphasise the complexity of the forces that impinge on the balance of the ecosystem in any individual's trilingual practices (see Aronin & Ó Laoire, 2004).

The classification of types of trilingual families that we introduced at the beginning of this book (see Figure 1.1, p. 5) can be seen as a recognition of some important patterns that occur in these ecosystems in mainly monolingual societies. At the same time, each of the families we described in Chapters 3–5 was unique in its linguistic and social configuration. Researchers such as Larissa Aronin and David Singleton have recognised our threegroup typology as a 'step ahead' classification 'beyond bilingualism' that attempts to explain trilingualism in the light of interacting factors (see Aronin & Singleton, 2012). In this chapter we have seen that multilingual communities share a similar variety and complexity in the histories that lie behind their current linguistic configuration. We have also seen that, in places like Luxembourg, that configuration may be changing rapidly in response to the impact of new patterns of migration. The stimulus for this book was an interest in the way globalisation is creating new patterns of trilingualism in formerly monolingual societies. But we must recognise that, at the same time, globalisation can also be a threat to linguistic diversity. That is the subject of the final section of this chapter.

Globalisation and the Rise of English

One outcome of globalisation has been the steady rise of English as the acknowledged global language. Many countries outside the English-speaking world have reacted to this development by giving greater priority to the teaching of English as a foreign language at school. Jasone Cenoz and Ulrike Jessner, who both have a long history of research into multilingualism, have collected reports of studies from authors in several European countries (see Cenoz & Jessner, 2000). The focus throughout is the influence of English as a factor in the growth of trilingualism in Europe. As we noted in our book, this is a subject of interest to many parents and educators at home, in the classroom and in the wider community. In bilingual societies, the impact of that has been to create new opportunities and support for trilingualism. This has been observed in trilingual education in the Basque Autonomous Community in the north of Spain, where teaching in Spanish and Basque in many schools has been complemented by teaching in English. Other examples in Europe include the Friesland province in the north of the Netherlands, where West Frisian is widely spoken alongside Dutch and the teaching of English is being introduced in an increasing number of schools. In Finland, the addition of English in schools has created an opportunity for the children of bilingual speakers of Swedish and Finnish to become trilingual. Annick De Houwer and Antje Wilton, who have edited the book *English in Europe Today: Sociocultural and Educational Perspectives* (2011), include empirical studies from several authors specialised in multilingualism. The emphasis is placed on the English language and how it interacts with other cultures and languages. Rather than highlighting the threats of English to other languages, the authors stress the sociolinguistic advantages of learning English as a second or third language.

Outside Europe, the international predominance of English has meant that ex-colonial societies such as Kenya have not rejected English as an official language even when an alternative, Kiswahili in this case, is also available. Many Kenyans speak a local ethnic language such as Gikuyu or Kikamba, the national language, Kiswahili, and English. In the past, three languages commonly coexisted: children in a town might use their mother tongue (an ethnic language) at home, Kiswahili when playing with friends and English at school or in church. Recent studies have indicated, however, that increasing numbers of young urban Kenyans are losing their mastery of their family's ethnic languages and focusing solely on Kiswahili and English. At national and international levels, the growth of a single dominant global language threatens trilingual capacity in many areas, even outside the mainly monolingual countries discussed in earlier chapters. One aim of this book is to describe how individual parents and families have attempted to counteract that tendency through their children's upbringing.

Summary

In this chapter we have discussed situations where children are raised in trilingual communities. While in monolingual societies only one language is used for every language domain, in trilingual societies three languages are spoken in different contexts, such as home, school and religious ceremonies. Here, speaking three languages is more likely to be seen as natural and to be encouraged by the majority of speakers. Children are more likely to grow up with a positive attitude towards trilingualism, which makes them feel proud and accepted. In monolingual societies, on the other hand, trilingualism can cause the opposite for children, who may feel marginalised and rejected as 'different'. Trilingual societies vary greatly in the historical basis of their current language heritage, and the nature of that history will influence how far residents share benign attitudes towards the various languages that are available to them. Even historically trilingual societies are becoming affected by more dominant languages, especially English, partly because of language contact, internet influence, education, media and (more generally) the economic pressures of globalisation. Some parents draw on multilingual schooling to support minority languages in an increasingly globalised world. In particular, European schools and international schools give a high priority to celebrating and producing active multilingualism. Other ways to support trilingualism are discussed in our concluding chapter.

7   Concluding Words

Introduction

In this final chapter of our book we will draw together ideas on how to support trilingual families. This must involve finding ways of tackling threats to using and maintaining three languages outside the family, at local, national and international level. There may be people in the community or even in a family who disapprove of trilingualism or who are worried that it could put too much pressure on children. In earlier chapters we have learned that, in predominantly monolingual societies, speaking languages other than the community language may be looked down on or stigmatised. This could cause trilingual families to feel uncomfortable using a minority language in public, especially if that language is regarded as 'low status'. We noted that this attitude was often reported in our research interviews and on the web forum.

When both the community and the family itself attribute positive values to minority languages, children are more likely to reach high levels of proficiency in two or even three languages and use them regularly when needed. This brings complementary positive elements to the person's overall development. Not only the technical skills of language use but also the cultural and social values associated with each language play a role in the child's multilingual character. In these circumstances, languages can be used without the threat that the community language will replace a minority language. In a multilingual environment where people speak various languages at different levels, mixing codes is almost normal, even natural. As a consequence, the emphasis on language accuracy is much less than is the case for people who grew up with only one main language. Even if the community supports multilingualism, parents still need strategies to pursue their goal, and such strategies are discussed in the next few pages.

Support for Trilingual Families

If parents use their home languages with their young babies, this will present structured language models for the children in more than one language. Many Group 1 families have found that OPOL (One Parent One Language) is a workable strategy that prevents language confusion (see Chapter 3). However, this may not be possible for bilingual or trilingual parents because they speak more than one language (see Chapters 4 and 5). Therefore additional strategies are needed to support all three languages so that they are used in the home more or less equally. Some parents and researchers suggest that the use of languages be split over a day, week or month, while others emphasise quality rather than quantity and explore the possibilities of intensive language exposure through watching television programmes and videos and reading books. In each case the opportunity can be taken to discuss the material (quite naturally) in the language in which it was presented.

In a recent publication, Annick De Houwer of the University of Erfurt in Germany discussed the principles underlying the development of a fluent use of language skills and fluency by young bilingual children before they start learning to read. She differentiated between multilingual children under the age of six who learnt two or more languages from birth and those who started a second or third language in an institutional setting such as a nursery or a day-care centre. Based on her own and other research, she stressed that the longer, the more intense and the more regular the exposure to each language, the more likely it is that a multilingual child will develop an appropriate level of language competence in each language for their age in terms of grammatical complexity, phonetic accuracy and vocabulary (see De Houwer, 2011).

Multilingual upbringing is usually determined by the perceived needs for children to be able to speak the community language and at the same time to develop an emotional connection with the parents' heritage languages and cultures, as well as to be able to communicate with relatives who do not know the community language. When bilingual and multilingual children use only the community language, harmonious communication within the family can be impeded. Research in general emphasises that early and structured exposure to a second or third language encourages the child to produce words and sentences in all three languages but it requires stamina, time and adventurous ideas.

When parents posted messages on the trilingualism.org website asking for advice, every case was considered separately, as there are no simple, universal answers. In this book we have highlighted three groups of trilingual families, but even within these groups there are variations. Often families move between different language constellations as they change their domicile, which was a common experience for trilingual families in our research and has frequently been reported by others. In most cases parents use one language with their young children, which usually is a native language (the language the parents grew up with during their formative years and which is culturally and emotionally their first language). Often the language choice comes naturally when a child is born. In our study and in contributions to the web forum, many parents in Group 1 families (those who speak one native language) linked their language choice to a sort of natural reflex. However, Group 2 parents (those who speak two native languages) described how they needed to make deliberate and conscious choices. These were often made against emotional and natural preferences but instead were based on convenience and language status. Group 3 parents (those who speak three or more languages individually) functioned similarly to Group 1 parents, in that they usually had one native language that was clearly the strongest and most accessible.

Other research has emphasised differences between bilingual and trilingual acquisition. For example, Gessica De Angelis of Trinity College Dublin has argued against research which views multilinguals as bilinguals with some extra languages. In fact, each language that is added results in a new language environment, which requires different language maintenance strategies. She summarised important factors that affect multilingualism in children and adults (see De Angelis, 2007). Some of these factors are the age of language acquisition, the amount of exposure to a particular language, the manner of acquisition (i.e. whether acquired at home or school) and active and passive use of languages. She also pointed out that these factors differ between learners acquiring a second language or a third language. This means that a trilingual person will experience challenges not known to bilingual speakers. For example, the time spent by trilingual learners using each of the three languages in their repertoire will usually be less than is the case for bilinguals and much less than for monolingual speakers. On the other hand, a child who is exposed to three languages may develop a language and cultural awareness that is richer and more differentiated than that of bilingual and monolingual learners.

Research has shown that the children of many potentially trilingual families, whatever their material circumstances, end up speaking only one language at an age-appropriate level. The worst scenario is when it looks as though none of the three languages is being developed properly. This can cause parents so much worry that some give up using minority languages with their children almost entirely. However, this is rare, and parents can feel reassured that the worst outcomes can be avoided. Researchers such as De Houwer and De Angelis have reviewed research which indicates that when structured and consistent opportunities are provided for learning more than one language, most infants and young children respond positively.

To support minority languages, some of the parents talked of sending their children to multilingual nurseries or schools, or employing multilingual nannies. But the starting point must be that the languages are used by parents with their children. Here are some questions to consider, based on the accounts we heard from the parents who have been quoted in this book, from the web discussion forum and from other authors in this field:

- Is cooking and helping in the kitchen associated with using a particular native language of one of the parents? Food and eating are emotionally resonant for most parents, and some dishes can best be described and discussed in the language of the country from which they come.
- Do the parents draw on the culture of lullabies and nursery rhymes with which they are most familiar, those of their own childhood?
- Does the family play common children's games in the forms associated with the parents' country of origin?

- Do the parents take advantage of any opportunities that occur for contact with other families who have children who speak the parents' native languages?
- Are there opportunities to visit the parents' home countries to experience the use of heritage languages and cultures at first hand?
- Do the families use Skype or other internet-based videoconferencing to contact grandparents and cousins in the parents' country of origin?
- Do parents provide their children with opportunities to read simple or advanced texts in their minority languages?
- Do members of the extended family, such as grandparents, send greeting cards, email invitations and letters in their heritage languages?
- Do parents use the internet or satellite television to provide regular access to the children's heritage languages and culture-specific programmes?

However, even though parents may wish fervently to use their heritage languages with their children, this is not always straightforward, especially when the children become older and leave the 'safe language environment' of the home. They will be exposed to other language models and may develop different ideas about language use from their parents and start to prefer the community language that is dominant in their peer group. This can be heartbreaking for some parents, as they are torn between, on the one hand, wanting their children to speak like local people and be accepted by them and, on the other hand, also wanting their children to speak their heritage language like the people in the parents' homeland. In a mainly monolingual society, bilingual and trilingual children may fail to develop some aspects of vocabulary in the language that is not used in the school context, making the school language the child's dominant and preferred language. Because of these language challenges, some parents have turned to the web and created blogs and forums. (For suggestions of useful further resources, see the appendices.)

English and Trilingualism

The influence of English often plays a considerable role in the development and maintenance of trilingualism. Although the global use of English has made it easy for people to communicate across borders, it has also brought discomfort to some speakers of minority languages. The use of English is so widespread as a global language that its presence is felt in almost all language domains. Many couples in trilingual families in our study communicated in English with each other and they worked in English-speaking environments. Knowledge of English has become a requirement for a career in an international environment due to its high status and position as a world language. It is not just English that has contributed to trilingualism worldwide over the centuries, but also Latin, Arabic, Spanish, French and Portuguese. However, the global dominance of English has now outplayed all previous world languages, to the extent that English as a third language (i.e. trilingualism) has emerged as a new research field. Historically bilingual communities have introduced English as a third language in school, such as

South Tyrol in Italy (Italian and German), Friesland in the Netherlands (West Frisian and Dutch) or the Basque Country in Spain (Basque and Spanish). It appears that education has played an important role in the spread of English, in particular in Europe, with governments introducing English as early as the preschool stage. About 90% of all pupils in the European Union learn English as a foreign language, and even in international multilingual schools English is often the medium of instruction. Parents in many trilingual families in Germany in our sample had enrolled their children in international English schools, even though some of them were not native speakers of English. For example, in Germany, Riitta, a Finnish mother, and her Dutch husband, Bert, took their children to an international English school. Although they were already struggling with Finnish, Dutch and German, they exposed their children to a fourth language.

Some researchers have criticised the use of English as a non-native language in a multilingual context, as it may interfere with the children's acquisition of the heritage languages. For example, Jasone Cenoz of the University of the Basque Country has looked at the effect of English as a third language in education in the Basque Country. In a recent report (Cenoz, 2000) she explained that although English as a foreign language is not very prominent in everyday life in the Basque Country, it is seen as prestigious and important in modern society. Up until the 1980s, French had been the preferred third language but then it was replaced by English, which is the case in many other countries. Parents are keen for their children to learn English as a third language after Basque and Spanish, because it can help them to communicate, travel and work across Europe and the world. English is also promoted in universities as enabling students to have access to wider knowledge and to get into more highly paid positions in banking and international business. In addition, teaching courses in English will also attract more foreign students and lecturers, boosting the international appeal of the university. However, there is also a trend at the University of the Basque Country that Basque has increasingly been adopted as the language of instruction over the last 10 years. So, despite the dominance of English in higher education, Basque has also enjoyed increasing popularity, partly because of the educational efforts in primary and secondary schooling and partly for political reasons. Nonetheless, English will become even more prominent, as foreign students who have this as the language they share with their potential tutors and fellow students seek to enrol in universities or colleges.

In our research, trilingual families in England seemed to find it even harder than families in Germany to maintain trilingualism, as English was also the language of the community, besides its global position in media, art and sciences. Most parents in England in our research had sent their children to English-speaking playgroups, nurseries or mainstream schools to provide their children with English in an academic environment, while the heritage languages were used only at home. Erum, a 37-year-old Persian-Farsi-speaking mother from Iran, said: 'I think it's better for the child if he gets used to the mother tongue, because he is fully immersed into an English environment at school, so [there is] no need to speak for him English at home'. The combination of the dominance, prestige and status of the English language seemed to have influenced most parents in England to send their children to mainstream schools. Even with young children, parents wanted their children to acquire English in nurseries or playgroups, because they were not using it at home. It meant, however, that many children who spent time away from home started to prefer to communicate in English, even with their parents.

Bringing Up Children Trilingually Against the Odds

One comment that is often heard is 'children learn a language without an effort'. That may be true for one language, but maintaining two languages is actually hard work in countries or communities with one dominant language, and even more effort is involved when there are three languages. In our research, parents commented on the challenges of trilingualism more often than its benefits, and many had never used their heritage languages with their children or had ceased to do so. In earlier chapters we showed that Group 2 families were struggling with raising their children trilingually, even though the potential was there, and that the challenge was even greater for Group 3 families. Most parents in these groups ended up using only one or in some instances two languages with their children. While trilingualism was less common in Group 2 and 3 families, some actually pursued trilingualism successfully 'against the odds'.

In our study of 70 trilingual families, only two Group 2 families and one Group 3 family used three languages with their children equally. All three families lived in Germany rather than England. In both Group 2 families, one of the parents spoke English as a native language. The children's learning of English was supported by their attending a multilingual school, where they also learned and spoke German. A third native language was spoken at home. For example, Ariana, who was a native speaker of German and English, was married to Dando, who had come from Italy. Despite the fact that Dando had lived in Germany for 15 years, he could barely speak German, as he worked in an environment where English was the main language. With their two boys, aged 5 and 10 years, the mother spoke English and German at home and the father spoke Italian. They sent their children to an international school, where they attended the Italian section for the main language of instruction, while English and German were taught as subject languages. In fact, Ariana said that 'My boys … primarily consider themselves Italians at the moment'. When Ariana was asked how they balanced the three languages she said:

> There is a continuing balancing act going on. Continued stimulation of the three main languages in school, with friends and in the environment keeps the balance.... I must remember not to mix the languages myself, because that can happen quite easily. I have to be the good example.

Ariana also listed the advantages of trilingualism in her family:

> Flexibility that allows us to live in different countries. Open mindedness and better understanding of another culture. The children are independent and fearless. A comparison made by a teacher: Many foreigners are sitting in a fish bowl, so the

sounds that come from outside are muted and not understood and they fear leaving their fishbowl, for lack of air. New languages are acquired more willingly.

There was also one Group 3 family in Germany trying to bring up their child trilingually 'against the odds'. These parents, who had a complex language history, used all three of their languages at home and in the community. The mother, Rasa, and her partner, Aras, spoke Russian and Lithuanian and the mother also spoke German as a native language, as she had moved to Germany when she was a teenager. Rasa used Russian and sometimes German and Aras Lithuanian with their 16-month-old son, Alex. This was a rare example, as both parents grew up in Lithuania, but Aras had gone to a Lithuanian-speaking school, whereas his partner had attended a Russian-speaking school. This meant that the father felt more attached to the Lithuanian language and culture, while his wife identified more with the Russian language. Although both parents spoke Russian and Lithuanian fluently, the father said that 'Rasa's mother tongue is Russian and mine is Lithuanian'.

Aras added: 'I try to speak Lithuanian and Rasa speaks Russian and in kindergarten Alex is exposed to German'. Although all three languages seemed to be used in a balanced way, there were worries that language delay might occur. Aras said: 'I'm a bit worried when he goes to kindergarten that his German is behind because we only speak Russian and Lithuanian at home'. Some people in the community also said that the child should learn more German and that three languages are too much. But Rasa was not too concerned: 'I'm not worried.... I know when I was small I grew up with two languages. When I went to kindergarten I couldn't speak any Lithuanian and it is not a problem for a child to learn a language.' (There is more information on this family in Chapter 5.)

Making a Success of It

Many people who are well known internationally for other reasons were multilingual, though that is not so well known. In science, for example, Albert Einstein, whose general theory of relativity revolutionised how we think of space and time, was born in Germany in 1879 but lived during his youth in Switzerland and Italy. He later migrated to the USA. Einstein was fluent in German, French, Italian and English.

In politics, Madeline Albright, a former Secretary of State of the USA, was born in the Czech Republic, where she attended a Swiss boarding school. When she was 11 years old she and her family moved to the USA. She is a fluent speaker of English, French and Czech. She also has effective speaking and reading skills in Polish, German and Russian.

Another major political figure with little-known trilingual competence was Franklin D. Roosevelt, the President of the USA from 1933 to 1945. Long before he led his country through the economic depression of the 1930s and through the Second World War, as a child he had developed proficiency in two other languages besides English – German and French, which he learned from German and French governesses.

A member of a political dynasty, though not herself a politician, Jacqueline Kennedy Onassis was another multilingual speaker in 20th-century public life in the USA. Her fluent command of Spanish and French and her ability to communicate in Italian and Polish may have been useful when she worked as a book editor and contributed as a patron of the arts. They were certainly exploited to the full during the presidential campaign of her husband, John F. Kennedy. It is reported that her mother had made sure that her daughters would learn to speak French by insisting that it was the only language allowed at the dinner table when she was a child.

Queen Silvia of Sweden may have a lower international profile but is an even more impressive linguist. She was born in Germany in 1943 and married King Carl XVI Gustaf of Sweden in 1976. At home she had learned German from her father and Portuguese from her Brazilian mother. Besides German, Portuguese and Swedish she also acquired French, Spanish and English.

In pop music, Shakira, the star of albums such as *Laundry Service*, was born in Colombia to a Spanish/Italian mother and Lebanese father. She learned to speak Spanish as her mother tongue and also acquired Arabic, Italian and Portuguese. She later moved to the USA, where she was not able to speak or write in English on arrival. Her best-known work as a singer/songwriter has been in English and Spanish.

Audrey Hepburn, the film actress, was born in Belgium to an Austrian father and a Dutch mother. When she was young, her mother's family links in the Netherlands and her father's work with a British company meant that the family often travelled between the three countries. Her parents separated when she was six, and she, her brothers and her mother lived first in England and then, during the Second World War, in the Netherlands. She later added fluent French, Spanish and Italian to the English and Dutch she had learned as a child.

The supermodel Claudia Schiffer, who has appeared on over 700 magazine covers, grew up in a small town by the Rhine as a monolingual speaker of German. She was spotted as a potential model at the age of 17 and spent a year in Paris, where she learned to speak fluent French, and subsequently settled in England, where she now speaks a 'lightly accented English'. She is still in demand for luxury fashion and fragrance houses. Claudia is fluent in German, English and French.

The tennis star Roger Federer, who has held the world number 1 position in his sport for longer than any other player, speaks four languages. He was born in Basel, Switzerland, to a Swiss father and a South African mother. He grew up in Switzerland close to the French and German borders and speaks Swiss German, German, French and English fluently.

The football star Cesc Fàbregas grew up in a small town north of Barcelona and spoke Spanish and Catalan from childhood. At the age of 16 he was recruited to the London Premier League team Arsenal, where he stayed for eight years, learning fluent English. As an adult in London he added French to his repertoire, claiming later that this was so that he could communicate with the many French speakers in the team led by Arsenal's French manager, Arsène Wenger.

Final Thoughts

As our experience of the world becomes more global through travel, internet and open borders, more people with different languages and cultures meet, live and work together. Societies with a monolingual history are experiencing an influx of new languages and cultures. Most have welcomed this development, though some may see it as a threat to their 'national identity'. Consequently, interest in the study of trilingualism has also increased, as parents and educators need and sometimes demand more information in order to meet the challenges of trilingualism at home, in school and in the community.

Our book offers a starting point for a broader understanding of the language practices of trilingual families with children in predominantly and historically monolingual countries. In general, trilingualism in Europe, as described in our book, is the result of globalisation and the recent political and geographical expansion of the European Union. But it does not stop there, as trilingualism has also become more common in America, Asia, Australia and Africa, which have enjoyed a long history of bilingualism. Working, studying and living in different countries has never been easier. It has created new opportunities and new challenges for parents with different national backgrounds and native languages to raise their children to be able to use their heritage languages.

Appendix: Resources for Trilingual Families with Children

Introduction

In this appendix you will find a brief guide to some of the books, articles and websites that may be of interest to parents and others who wish to explore issues related to trilingualism further after reading this book. In recent years there has been a slight increase in the number of books and published articles that deal with acquiring more than two languages. Parents in trilingual families often live in comparative language isolation, as there are few households with exactly the same language combination living close to them. It is commonly impossible for new parents in this situation to turn to their own parents or extended family for advice because they themselves do not share the same trilingual context. So in the digital age the first place where many parents look for information about trilingualism is the internet. There is now extensive advice on multilingualism, but it is often difficult to judge what it is based on. In addition, it may not be clear how any insights might apply to one's own situation because almost every family functions differently in terms of the languages spoken, the language constellation, age of parents, age of children and so on. Personal accounts are fascinating and can be helpful, but it would be wrong to just try to copy 'successful' trilingual families. In the research on which this book is based we learned that it is not possible to give universal answers to parents who seek help and support for their trilingual children. In this guide we try to make clear what specific help each resource may offer.

Websites

- **Multilingualliving.com** – 'Because global communication begins at home'. This site was founded in 2004 by Corey Heller. It was first named Bilingual/Bicultural Family Network but later changed to Multilingual Living. The starting point was Corey's interest as the mother of a multilingual family. She was born in the USA and her husband in Germany. The site is designed for bilingual as well as for trilingual families. There are articles on trilingualism and the active discussion forum has many trilingual topics. Contributors include parents, researchers and teachers. The founder's aim was that the site should be 'a place where parents raising children in more than one language and culture can find inspiration, tools, advice, wisdom and support! It is about living multilingually, in each and every way possible.'

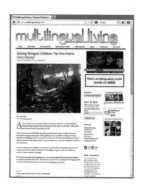

- **Multilingualchildren.org** – Multilingual Children's Association (MCA). This is the website of the Multilingual Children's Association, which is based in San Francisco. It was founded by Christina Bosemark, who brought up her two daughters in California to speak English, Swedish and Spanish. The site focuses on bilingual issues, but the active Discussion Forum has some threads on trilingual families. It aims to be 'your web-guide to raising multilingual children … an entire site dedicated to kids growing up with multiple languages – expert advice and real world wisdom, parent discussions, tips, resource directory, articles and more.'

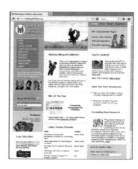

- **Trilingualism.org** – Growing up with three languages and cultures. This site was established by the first author of this book in 2003. Andreas, who was brought up in Germany, and his Finnish wife have lived in Germany and Finland with their two children and are now settled in England. This website aims to support trilinguals, parents, teachers and others to develop a better understanding of trilingualism in school, family and the wider community. It has a continuing Discussion Forum and a stronger research emphasis than the two previous sites, with publications, abstracts and presentations relating to Andreas's own research and links to reports of studies by other researchers in the field of trilingualism.

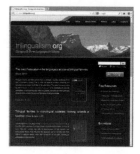

Blogs on Multilingual Issues

- Madalena Cruz-Ferreira is Portuguese, married to a Swede, living in Singapore and working (mostly) in English. She has three trilingual children (studied and celebrated in her best-known book, which is included in the list of books below). Her personal blog is informed by a mix of personal experience in a trilingual family and professional expertise as a linguist, educator and researcher (http:// beingmultilingual.blogspot.co.uk).

- Jan (who is German) and Souad (who blogs as BabelMum) speak German, French, English and Arabic between them and live in England. In the babelkid blog, which they set up in 2007, they describe episodes in their daily life with their trilingual (quadrilingual?) children with humour and a constant interest in their language (http://www.babelkid.net).

- Trilingual Family Chinese mum + French dad + Australian daughter: A Chinese Mum and a French Dad decided to move to Australia in 2008, where their first baby girl was born four years later. Nicolas, her dad, speaks French, English and reasonable Mandarin Chinese, while the mum speaks Mandarin Chinese, fluent English and pretty fluent French as well as two Chinese dialects. This blog on raising trilingual children is updated regularly and includes an archive, a blog-roll and links to other useful websites related to multilingualism (http://trilingualfamily.wordpress.com).

Online Research Reports

- 'Issues surrounding trilingual families: Children with simultaneous exposure to three languages' (http://zif.spz.tu-darmstadt.de/jg-05-1/beitrag/barron.htm) reports a survey conducted by Suzanne Barron-Hauwaert with 10 trilingual families across Europe. She was interested in how the three languages co-existed in each family, what choices the parents made regarding their children's education, how the families dealt with language mixing, and how they defined themselves culturally and linguistically.

- 'Trilingual first language acquisition: Exploration of a linguistic "miracle"' (http:// www.bbk.ac.uk/lachouette/chou31/Dewael31.pdf) describes the wonderment and fascination of Jean-Marc Dewaele as he charts the early trilingual development of his daughter Livia growing up in London and learning Dutch, French and English simultaneously.

- 'One? ¿Dos? Drei! A study of code switching in child trilingualism' (http://ir.uiowa. edu/etd/484) reports the doctoral research completed in 2010 by Elena Davidiak. She describes two girls who were aged six and nine years when the study began and were living in New York. Their parents were native speakers of German and Spanish with English as the language they used for education and in the wider community.

Trilingual speakers often switch between languages ('code switching'). Elena examined the extent to which the girls made such switches and what appeared to cause them to do so in particular situations. Was it only because of deficiencies in the vocabulary in one of the languages, or were there other causes? She found that even at this age they used 'code switching' for various other reasons, such as to refer to a specific person or to include or exclude someone from the conversation or because they had changed who they were talking to or what they were talking about. Like everything else to do with language, it did not stay still. The amount of switching and the reasons for it changed dynamically as the children got older and always reflected the age difference between the sisters and the relationship between them.

- 'The nature of two trilingual children's utterances: Growing up with Croatian, English and German' (https://ueaeprints.uea.ac.uk/34212) reports doctoral research completed in 2011 by Ksenija Corinna Ivir-Ashworth. She studied language mixing by two siblings aged one and three years. Those who would like to find out more about how very young children mix languages within words and within sentences may find Chapter 6 of particular interest. This describes a technical analysis of how the two trilingual children spoke in different situations.

Books from Parents in Trilingual Families

- *Growing up with Three Languages: Birth to Eleven*. Published by Multilingual Matters (2008). Xiao-lei Wang was born and grew up in China and now lives with her Swiss husband and their two children in the USA. This book is based on 11 years of observation of the children's development in a family where English, French and Chinese are spoken daily. The book explains how the children have negotiated their three languages and cultures and have developed a unique identity. She summarises the overarching goal of the book as 'to help parents see the possibilities for raising children with three languages when parents are the major source of the heritage language input, and make efforts to preserve their heritage language(s) starting at the family level'.

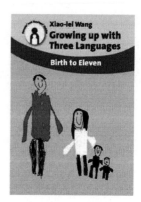

- *Learning to Read and Write in the Multilingual Family*. Published by Multilingual Matters (2011). Xiao-lei Wang wrote this book in response to parents of trilingual children who had read her earlier book, mentioned above. Parents asked how multilingual children could learn to read and write in three languages. In this book, Xia-lei discusses multi-literacy in multilingual learners during different stages, from infancy to adolescence. The book also gives practical advice to parents in terms of strategies and language practices.

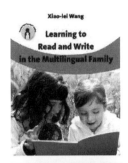

- *Early Trilingualism: A Focus on Questions*. Published by Multilingual Matters (2006). Julia Barnes explains in detail how a trilingual young girl, Jenny, acquired English with limited exposure. The family lives in the Basque Country of Spain, where Basque and Spanish are spoken. The mother used English with Jenny and the father spoke in Basque, while Spanish was mainly heard through television, a caregiver and the community. This academic book provides a meticulous account of the language practices of a trilingual family.

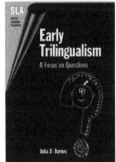

- *Three Is a Crowd? Acquiring Portuguese in a Trilingual Environment*. Published by Multilingual Matters (2006). Madalena Cruz-Ferreira, whose blog was listed earlier, describes and analyses her three children's language development, with a particular focus on their use of Portuguese, in a multilingual family and social environment in which they also learnt Swedish and English. In her book, Madalena explores themes such as balancing culture and identity, language input and language management, acquiring a third language and becoming multilingual.

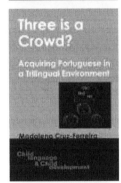

- *Raising Multilingual Children: Foreign Language Acquisition and Children*. Published by Bergin & Garvey (2001). Tracey Tokuhama-Espinosa, who was born in the USA, lives in Ecuador, where she has brought up three multilingual children in English, Spanish, German and French. Her observations have suggested that parents who are successful in bringing up their children multilingually often take advantage of third-language opportunities from birth, when the brain seems to process new languages more easily than in adults. Her experience has led to her strong support for the One Parent One Language strategy, which she says has yielded the best results.

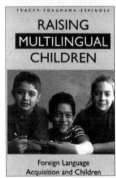

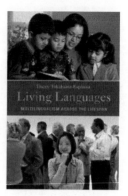

- *Living Languages: Multilingualism Across the Lifespan.* Published by Praeger Publishers (2008). Tracey Tokuhama-Espinosa's recent book on multilingualism reflects on over 15 years of research, including seeing her own multilingual children growing up. The book is grounded in the reported experiences of hundreds of multilingual families and teachers in 15 countries. Tracey aimed to write a book that 'helps parents to sail through the heavy seas of doubt that can accompany this multilingual adventure at different stages of the voyage'.

Multilingual Education

- *Pathways to Multilingualism: Evolving Perspectives on Immersion Education.* Published by Multilingual Matters (2008). In this book the editors, Tara Williams Fortune and Diane J. Tedick, aim to highlight ways in which multilingualism can be supported through immersion education. This is a strategy in which some school subjects are taught in a minority language rather than all being taught in the majority language of the community. The chapter authors draw their conclusions from theoretical perspectives, empirical studies and research reviews linked to language development in immersion programmes.

- *Multilingual Learning: Stories from Schools and Communities in Britain.* Published by Trentham Books (2007). The editors, Jean Conteh, Peter Martin and Leena Helavaara Robertson, call for a rethink of how both mainstream and community schools respond to the multilingual potential of their students. The theme is illustrated with chapters from a number of authors in the field, who tell the stories of children or schools that they know well.

- *Imagining Multilingual Schools: Languages in Education and Glocalization.* Published by Multilingual Matters (2006). Ofelia Garcia, Tove Skutnabb-Kangas and Maria E. Torres-Guzman have edited this book, which explores the pedagogical, socio-educational and socio-political aspects of multilingual schools. Chapters include 'Imagining Multilingual Education in France', 'Attitudes Towards Language Learning in Different Linguistic Models of the Basque Autonomous Community' and 'The Long Road to Multilingual Schools in Botswana'.

- *Encyclopedia of Language and Education, Vol. 5: Bilingual Education.* Published by Springer (2010). Jim Cummins and Nancy H. Hornberger, who edited this volume, are leading scholars in the field. Chapter authors reflect on key policy issues and socio-political challenges facing proponents of bilingual education across the world. There are chapters on bilingual education in trilingual settings, such as Singapore, and on different approaches to the development of language proficiency in multilingual education.

- *Towards Multilingual Education: Basque Education Research from an International Perspective.* Published by Multilingual Matters (2009). Jason Cenoz, a leading researcher in the field of multilingualism, explains the development of multilingual forms of education. Themes include, for example, third-language learning and instruction through a third language, learning through a minority language, and the influence of bilingualism on the learning of a third language. The age factor in language learning is also covered. The book is mainly based on a case study of the Basque Country, but is also relevant for other contexts and multilingual communities.

Additional Academic Books on Multilingualism

- *Trilingualism in Family, School and Community.* Published by Multilingual Matters (2004). The editors of this book, Charlotte Hoffmann and Jehannes Ytsma, have drawn together research from well known authors around the world. The studies described in the book focus on trilingualism as distinguished from bilingualism and cover areas such as trilingual language use, language policy and education, as well as the pros and cons of trilingualism. The experience of being trilingual and of raising children trilingually must have given a personal perspective to the editing process.

- *Third or Additional Language Acquisition.* Published by Multilingual Matters (2007). Gessica De Angelis has worked as an Italian language teacher and researcher in different countries for many years. Although written in an academic style, this book is easy to read and offers an up-to-date overview of research conducted in areas such as cognitive development in multilingual speakers, third-language acquisition and multilingual speech production. The book looks beyond bilingualism by exploring the challenges when a third or fourth language is acquired.

- *The Multilingual Mind: Issues Discussed By, For, and About People Living With Many Languages.* Published by Praeger (2003). This semi-formal book includes chapters from 11 different authors, such as Suzanne Barron-Hauwaert, Nicola Küpelikilinc and Tracey Tokuhama-Espinosa. The book is written for parents and others interested in multilingualism. The main themes relate to schooling, multi-literacy, identity and generally children's trilingualism. Tracey, the editor, concludes the book with her own words: 'My hope is that each answer here breeds a new series of questions, which will in turn bring further attention to the rich depths of the multilingual mind'.

- *An Introduction to Bilingual Development.* Published by Multilingual Matters (2009). In this introductory textbook Annick De Houwer describes the development of children who grow up hearing two languages from birth. Many children in trilingual families share the early experience of the children featured in this book. Themes include, for example, bilingual learning in context, bilingual first-language acquisition and preschool and beyond.

References and Further Reading

Chapter 1

Barron-Hauwaert, S. (2000) Issues surrounding trilingual families: Children with simultaneous exposure to three languages. *Zeitschrift für Interkulturelle Fremdsprachenunterricht* 5 (1), 1–13 (http://zif.spz.tu-darmstadt.de/jg-05-1/beitrag/barron.htm).

Braun, A. (2006) The effect of sociocultural and linguistic factors on the language use of parents in trilingual families in England and Germany. Doctoral dissertation, University of Bedfordshire (http://uobrep.openrepository.com/uobrep/handle/10547/279452).

Dewaele, J-M. (2000) Trilingual first language acquisition: exploration of a linguistic 'miracle'. *LaChouette* 31, 41–45 (http://www.bbk.ac.uk/lachouette/chou31/Dewael31.pdf).

European Commission. Official EU languages, at http://ec.europa.eu/languages/languages-of-europe/eu-languages_en.htm.

Guardian (2012) David Cameron attacks Ed Miliband's immigration plans. 14 December, at http://www.guardian.co.uk/uk/2012/dec/14/david-cameron-ed-miliband-immigration

Office for National Statistics. International migrants in England and Wales 2011, at http://www.ons.gov.uk/ons/dcp171776_290335.pdf.

Omniglot. Raising bilingual children: The different methods to success, at http://www.omniglot.com/language/articles/bilingualkids4.htm.

Statistisches Bundesamt. Bevölkerung und Erwerbstätigkeit [national statistics for Germany 2011], at https://www.destatis.de/DE/Publikationen/Thematisch/Bevoelkerung/MigrationIntegration/AuslaendBevoelkerung2010200117004.pdf?__blob=publicationFile

Chapter 2

Web-based sources

Barron-Hauwaert, S. (2000) Issues surrounding trilingual families: Children with simultaneous exposure to three languages. *Zeitschrift für Interkulturelle Fremdsprachenunterricht* 5 (1), 1–13 (http://zif.spz.tu-darmstadt.de/jg-05-1/beitrag/barron.htm)

Benson-Cohen, C. (2005) Oral competence and OPOL: Factors affecting success. *Bilingual Family Newsletter* 22 (4), 4–5 (http://www.bilingualfamilynewsletter.com/download.php?filetosend=BFN%2022-4.pdf).

Davidiak, E. (2010) One¿ ¿Dos¿ Drei! A study of code switching in child trilingualism (http://ir.uiowa.edu/etd/484).

Ivir-Ashworth, K.C. (2011) The nature of two trilingual children's utterances: Growing up with Croatian, English and German. Doctoral dissertation, University of East Anglia (https://ueae-prints.uea.ac.uk/34212).

Kovács, A.M. and Mehler, J. (2009) Cognitive gains in 7-month-old bilingual infants. *PNAS* 106 (16), 6556–6560 (http://www.pnas.org/content/early/2009/04/13/0811323106.full.pdf).

Perry, S. (2008) The bilingual brain (http://www.brainfacts.org/Sensing-Thinking-Behaving/Language/Articles/2008/The-Bilingual-Brain).

Petitto, L-A. and Dunbar, K.N. (2009) Educational neuroscience: New discoveries from bilingual brains, scientific brains, and the educated mind. *Mind, Brain, and Education* 3 (4), 185–197 (http://www.ncbi.nlm.nih.gov/pmc/articles/PMC3338206).

Books and book chapters

Baker, C. (2000) *A Parent's and Teacher's Guide to Bilingualism* (2nd edition). Clevedon: Multilingual Matters.

Baker, C. (2011) *Foundations of Bilingual Education and Bilingualism* (5th edition). Bristol: Multilingual Matters.

Barnes, J. (2006) *Early Trilingualism: A Focus on Questions*. Clevedon: Multilingual Matters.

Barron-Hauwaert, S. (2004) *Language Strategies for Bilingual Families: The One-Parent-One-Language Approach*. Clevedon: Multilingual Matters.

Barron-Hauwaert, S. (2011) *Bilingual Siblings*. Bristol: Multilingual Matters.

Braun, A. (2008) A sociocultural perspective on the language practices of trilingual families in England and Germany. In R. Temmerman, J. Darquennes and F. Boers (eds) *Multilingualism and Applied Comparative Linguistics. Vol. 2: Cross-Cultural Communication, Translation Studies and Multilingual Terminology* (pp. 44–63). Newcastle: Cambridge Scholars Press.

Cenoz, J. (2000) Research on multilingual acquisition. In J. Cenoz and U. Jessner (eds) *English in Europe: The Acquisition of a Third Language* (pp. 39–53). Clevedon: Multilingual Matters.

Cummins, J. (1981) *Bilingualism and Minority Language Children*. Ontario: Ontario Institute for Studies in Education.

De Houwer, A. (2004) Trilingual input and children's language use in trilingual families in Flanders. In C. Hoffmann and J. Ytsma (eds) *Trilingualism in Family, School and Community* (pp. 118–135). Clevedon: Multilingual Matters.

De Houwer, A. (2009) *An Introduction to Bilingual Development*. Bristol: Multilingual Matters.

Gathercole, V.C.M. (2002) Grammatical gender in bilingual and monolingual children: A Spanish morphosyntactic distinction. In D. Kimbrough Oller and R.E. Eilers (eds) *Language and Literacy in Bilingual Children* (pp. 207–219). Clevedon: Multilingual Matters.

Herdina, P. and Jessner, U. (2002) *A Dynamic Model of Multilingualism: Perspectives of Change in Psycholinguistics*. Clevedon: Multilingual Matters.

Hoffmann, C. and Ytsma, J. (eds) (2004) *Trilingualism in Family, School and Community*. Clevedon: Multilingual Matters.

Meisel, J.M. (ed.) (1994) *Bilingual First Language Acquisition: French and German Grammatical Development*. Amsterdam: John Benjamins.

Meisel, J.M. (ed.) (2011) *First and Second Language Acquisition: Parallels and Differences* (Cambridge Textbooks in Linguistics). Cambridge: Cambridge University Press.

Pearson, B.Z. (2008) *Raising a Bilingual Child*. New York: Living Language.

Ronjat, J. (1913) *Le development du langage observe chez un enfant bilingue*. Paris: Champion.

Tokuhama-Espinosa, T. (ed.) (2003) *The Multilingual Mind: Issues Discussed by, For, and About People Living With Many Languages*. London: Praeger.

Wang, X-L. (2008) *Growing Up With Three Languages – Birth to Eleven*. Bristol: Multilingual Matters.

Journal articles and conference papers

Bialystok, E. (1999) Cognitive complexity and attentional control in the bilingual mind. *Child Development* 70, 636–644.

Braun, A. and Cline, T. (2010) Trilingual families in monolingual societies: Working towards a typology. *International Journal of Multilingualism* 7 (2), 110–127.

Clyne, M., Hunt, R. and Isaakidis, T. (2004) Learning a community language as a third language. *International Journal of Multilingualism* 1, 33–52.

Cummins, J. (1976) The influence of bilingualism on cognitive growth: A synthesis of research findings and explanatory hypotheses. *Working Papers on Bilingualism* 9, 1 –43.

Cummins, J. (1979) Linguistic interdependence and the educational development of bilingual children. *Review of Educational Research* 49, 222–251.

Gorter, D. (2006) Introduction: The study of the linguistic landscape as a new approach to multilingualism. *International Journal of Multilingualism* 3 (1), 1–6.

Kamwangamalu, N.M. (2001) The language planning situation in South Africa. *Current Issues in Language Planning* 2 (4), 361–445. (Monograph.)

Kovelman, I. and Petitto, L-A. (2002) Bilingual babies' maturational and linguistic milestones as a function of their age of first exposure to two languages. Poster presented at the Conference for the Society for Neuroscience, Orlando, FL.

Lasagabaster, D. (1998) The threshold hypothesis applied to three languages in contact at school. *International Journal of Bilingual Education and Bilingualism* 1 (2), 119–133.

Petitto, L-A. (2009) New discoveries from the bilingual brain and mind across the life span: Implications for education. *Mind, Brain, and Education* 3 (4), 185–197.

Verhoeven, L.T. and Boeschoten, H.E. (1986) First language acquisition in a second language submersion environment. *Applied Psycholinguistics* 7 (3), 241–255.

Chapter 3

Barnes, J.D. (2006) *Early Trilingualism: A Focus on Questions.* Clevedon: Multilingual Matters.

Barron-Hauwaert, S. (2004) *Language Strategies for Bilingual Families: The One-Parent-One-Language Approach.* Clevedon: Multilingual Matters.

Cruz-Ferreira, M. (2006) *Three Is a Crowd? Acquiring Portuguese in a Trilingual Environment.* Clevedon: Multilingual Matters.

De Angelis, G. (2007) *Third or Additional Language Acquisition.* Clevedon: Multilingual Matters.

Lambert, W.E. (1987) The effects of bilingual and bicultural experiences on children's attitudes and social perspectives. In P. Homel, M. Palij and D. Aaronson (eds) *Childhood Bilingualism: Aspects of Linguistic Cognitive and Social Development* (pp. 192–221). Hillsdale, NJ: Lawrence Erlbaum.

Lasagabaster, D. and Huguet, A. (2007) *Multilingualism in European Bilingual Contexts: Language Use and Attitudes.* Clevedon: Multilingual Matters.

Chapter 4

Baker, C. (2011) *Foundations of Bilingual Education and Bilingualism* (5th edition). Bristol: Multilingual Matters.

Benson-Cohen, C. (2005) Oral competence and OPOL: Factors affecting success. *Bilingual Family Newsletter* 22 (4), 4–5 (http://www.bilingualfamilynewsletter.com/download.php?filetosend=BFN%20 22-4.pdf).

De Angelis, G. and Dewaele, J.M. (2011) *New Trends in Crosslinguistic Influence and Multilingualism Research.* Bristol: Multilingual Matters.

Küpelikilinc, N. (2003) What, you speak only one language!¿ A trilingual family's story. In T. Toku-hama-Espinosa (ed.) *The Multilingual Mind* (pp. 151–162). London: Praeger.
Wikipedia. Plautdietsch, or Mennonite Low German language, at http://en.wikipedia.org/wiki/Plaut-dietsch_language.
Wang, X.-L. (2008) *Growing Up With Three Languages: Birth to Eleven*. Bristol: Multilingual Matters.
Wang, X.-L. (2011) *Learning to Read and Write in the Multilingual Family*. Bristol: Multilingual Matters.

Chapter 5

Aronin, L. and Hufeisen, B. (2009) *The Exploration of Multilingualism*. Amsterdam: John Benjamins.
Cenoz, J. and Jessner, U. (eds) (2000) *English in Europe: The Acquisition of a Third Language*. Clevedon: Multilingual Matters.
De Houwer, A. and Wilton, A. (2011) *English in Europe Today: Sociocultural and Educational Perspectives*. Amsterdam: John Benjamins.
Garcia, O., Skutnabb-Kangas, T. and Guzman, M.E. (2006) *Imagining Multilingual Schools: Languages in Education and Glocalization*. Clevedon: Multilingual Matters.

Chapter 6

Web-based sources

Benson-Cohen, C. (2005) Oral competence and OPOL: Factors affecting success. *Bilingual Family News-letter* 22 (4), 4–5 (http://www.bilingualfamilynewsletter.com/download.php¿filetosend=BFN%20 22-4.pdf).
Braun, A. (2011) Trilingual families of the global village – and what about the grandparents¿ Paper presented at the Seventh International Conference on Third Language Acquisition and Multilin-gualism, Warsaw, Poland (at http://www.trilingualism.org).
European Commission (Eurostat) Foreign language learning statistics, at http://epp.eurostat.ec.europa. eu/statistics_explained/index.php/Foreign_language_learning_statistics.
FMKS (Frühe Mehrsprachigkeit an Kitas und Schulen e.V – Association for Early Multilingualism in Day Nurseries and Schools), at http://www.fmks-online.de.
Michieka, M. (2012) Language maintenance and shift among Kenyans. In B. Connell and N. Rolle (eds) *Selected Proceedings of the 41st Annual Conference on African Linguistics* (pp. 164–170). Somerville, MA: Cascadilla Proceedings Project (http://www.lingref.com/cpp/acal/41/paper2746.pdf).
Mueller, M. (2012) Sri Lanka launches plan to become trilingual nation. Asia Foundation, 28 March, at http://asiafoundation.org/in-asia/2012/03/28/sri-lanka-launches-plan-to-become-trilingual-nation.
Schola Europaea. European schools, at http://www.eursc.eu.
Wachira, A.W. (2006) Multilingualism in Kenya: Focus on language use and its implications. *Internet-Zeitschrift für Kulturwissenschaften* 16, at http://www.inst.at/trans/16Nr/03_2/wachira16.htm.
Wikipedia. Languages of Luxembourg, at http://en.wikipedia.org/wiki/Languages_of_Luxembourg.
Wikipedia. Languages of Singapore, at http://en.wikipedia.org/wiki/Languages_of_Singapore.

Journal articles

Auleear Owodally, A.M. (2012) Juggling languages: A case study of preschool teachers' language choices and practices in Mauritius. *International Journal of Multilingualism* 9 (3), 235–256.
Banda, F. (2009) Critical perspectives on language planning and policy in Africa: Accounting for the notion of multilingualism. *Stellenbosch Papers in Linguistics* 38, 1–11.

Braun, A. (2012) Language maintenance in trilingual families – a focus on grandparents. *International Journal of Multilingualism* 9 (4), 423–436.

Brohy, C. (2005) Trilingual education in Switzerland. *International Journal of the Sociology of Language* 171, 133–148.

Ceginskas, V. (2010) Being 'the strange one' or 'like everybody else': School education and the negotiation of multilingual identity. *International Journal of Multilingualism* 7 (3), 211–224.

Grin, F. (1995) The economics of language competence: a research project of the Swiss National Science Foundation. *Journal of Multilingual and Multicultural Development* 16, 227–231.

Grosjean, F. (1985) The bilingual as a competent but specific speaker-hearer. *Journal of Multilingual and Multicultural Development*, 6(6): 467–77.

Hayden, M.C. and Thompson, J.J. (1997) Student perspectives on international education: A European dimension. *Oxford Review of Education* 23 (4), 459–478.

Kirsch, C. (2006) Young children learning languages in a multilingual context. *International Journal of Multilingualism* 3 (4), 258–279.

Kreindler, I., Bensoussan, M., Avinor, E. and Bram, C. (1995) Circassian Israelis: Multilingualism as a way of life. *Language, Culture and Curriculum* 8 (2 – special issue: Multilingualism and language learning), 149–162.

Savvides, N. (2008) The European dimension in education: Exploring pupils' perceptions at three European schools. *Journal of Research in International Education* 7 (3), 304–326.

Sinha, S. (2009) Code switching and code mixing among Oriya trilingual children – a study. *Language in India* 9, 274–283.

Books and book chapters

Aronin, L. and Ó Laoire, M. (2004) Exploring multilingualism in cultural contexts: Towards a notion of multilinguality. In C. Hoffmann and J. Ytsma (eds) *Trilingualism in Family, School and Community* (pp. 11–30). Clevedon: Multilingual Matters.

Aronin, L. and Singleton, D. (2012) *Multilingualism*. Amsterdam: John Benjamins.

Benson, C. (2004) Trilingualism in Guinea-Bissau and the question of instructional language. In C. Hoffman and J. Ytsma (eds) *Trilingualism in Family, School and Community* (pp. 166–184). Clevedon: Multilingual Matters.

Braun, A. (2011) The role of education in the language practices of trilingual families. In C. Varcasia (ed.) *Becoming Multilingual: Language Learning and Language Policy Between Attitudes and Identities* (p. 113–134). Bern: Peter Lang.

Cenoz, J. and Jessner, U. (eds) (2000) *English in Europe: The Acquisition of a Third Language*. Clevedon: Multilingual Matters.

Conteh, J., Martin, P. and Roberstson, L.H. (eds) (2007) *Multilingual Learning: Stories from Schools and Communities in Britain*. Stoke-on-Trent: Trentham Books.

Cummins, J. and Hornberger, N.H. (eds) (2010) *Encyclopedia of Language and Education, Vol. 5: Bilingual Education*. New York: Springer.

De Houwer, A. and Wilton, A. (2011) *English in Europe Today: Sociocultural and Educational Perspectives*. Amsterdam: John Benjamins.

Ferreira-Cruz, M. (2006) *Three Is a Crowd? Acquiring Portuguese in a Trilingual Environment*. Clevedon: Multilingual Matters.

Fortune, T.W. and Tedick, D.J. (eds) (2008) *Pathways to Multilingualism: Evolving Perspectives on Immersion Education*. Clevedon: Multilingual Matters.

Garcia, O., Skutnabb-Kangas, T. and Guzman, M.E. (2006) *Imagining Multilingual Schools: Languages in Education and Glocalization*. Clevedon: Multilingual Matters.

Suils, J. and Huguet, A. (2001) The Occitan speech community of the Aran Valey. In M.T. Turell (ed.) *Multilingualism in Spain* (pp. 144–164). Clevedon: Multilingual Matters.

Chapter 7

Barron-Hauwaert, S. (2004) *Language Strategies for Bilingual Families: The One-Parent-One-Language Approach*. Clevedon: Multilingual Matters.

Cenoz, J. (2000) Research on multilingual acquisition. In J. Cenoz and U. Jessner (eds) *English in Europe: The Acquisition of a Third Language* (pp. 39–53). Clevedon: Multilingual Matters.

Cenoz, J. (2009) *Towards Multilingual Education: Basque Educational Research from an International Perspective*. Bristol: Multilingual Matters.

Cenoz, J. and Jessner, U. (eds) (2000) *English in Europe: The Acquisition of a Third Language*. Clevedon: Multilingual Matters.

Crystal, D. (2003) *English as a Global Language*. Cambridge: Cambridge University Press.

De Angelis, G. (2007) *Third or Additional Language Acquisition*. Clevedon: Multilingual Matters.

De Houwer, A. (2011) The speech of fluent child bilinguals. In P. Howell and J.V. Borsel (eds) *Multilingual Aspects of Fluency Disorders* (pp. 3–23). Bristol: Multilingual Matters.

De Houwer, A. and Wilton, A. (2011) *English in Europe Today: Sociocultural and Educational Perspectives*. Amsterdam: John Benjamins.

Tokuhama-Espinosa, T. (2001) *Raising Multilingual Children: Foreign Language Acquisition and Children*. London: Bergin & Garvey.

Wang, X-L. (2008) *Growing Up With Three Languages – Birth to Eleven*. Bristol: Multilingual Matters.

Index